D1318070

Pontiac, Michigan

ETHOLOGY AND PSYCHIATRY

156
E84

Ethology and Psychiatry

Edited by *Norman F. White*

FROM THE CLARENCE M. HINCKS
MEMORIAL LECTURES,
HELD AT McMASTER UNIVERSITY,
1970

Published for the
Ontario Mental Health Foundation
by University of Toronto Press

© University of Toronto Press 1974
Toronto and Buffalo
Printed in Canada
ISBN (cloth) 0-8020-3309-1
ISBN (paper) 0-8020-3312-1
LC 73-78941

Contents

039763

Contributors

COLIN G. BEER university lecturer in Zoology, and Fellow of New College, Oxford University

JOHN HURRELL CROOK reader in Ethology, Psychology Department, Bristol University

IRVEN DEVORE professor of Anthropology, Harvard University

DAVID HAMBURG professor, Department of Psychiatry, Stanford University School of Medicine

ERNST W. HANSEN professor, Department of Psychology, Rutgers University

HARRY F. HARLOW professor, Department of Psychology, and Director of the Primate Laboratory, University of Wisconsin

SUZANNE D. HILL* Department of Psychology, Louisiana State University at New Orleans

ROBERT A. HINDE Royal Society Research Professor, MRC Unit on the Development and Integration of Behaviour, University of Cambridge

I. CHARLES KAUFMAN professor of Psychiatry, University of Colorado Medical Center

MELVIN J. KONNER* post-doctoral fellow, Foundations Fund for Research in Psychiatry, Harvard University

† DANIEL S. LEHRMAN formerly professor of Psychology, and Director of the Institute of Animal Behavior, Rutgers University

PETER MARLER professor of Zoology, The Rockefeller University

WILLIAM A. MASON professor of Psychology, Department of Psychology, University of California (Davis)

JAY S. ROSENBLATT professor of Psychology, Director of the Institute of Animal Behavior, Rutgers University, and practicing psychoanalyst

CURTIS E. THOMSEN* Department of Psychology, Tulane University

NORMAN F. WHITE* Department of Psychology, McMaster University

* Not participants in the meeting
† See page xi

Preface

Psychiatry and ethology are both fields which hold a good deal of interest for biological scientists, the general public, and all workers in the 'helping professions.' Where their ideas intersect, therefore, one could expect the literature to show some comment and scholarly examination of the concerns they share. That this has not occurred to any great extent is an anomaly for which this book attempts a partial remedy. Perhaps the explanation is best sought in the evolution of each discipline, a theme consistent with the main burden of the chapters that follow. We may presume, because of the overlap of their intellectual territories, that each field can enrich and support the other, but the articles presented here focus on the increasingly important contributions made in only one direction — from ethology to psychiatry.

It is not a book on ethology — there are now a number of excellent ones available — but is intended as a preliminary guide to the reader in his further excursions into either field. The need for such guidance is clear. From the popular press has come, over the past few years, an increasing volume of books and articles which draw on animal studies and purport to be scientific explanations of human behaviour. It has never been exactly clear to the layman, or the scientist, what to make of animal data. Public ambivalence has ranged from the stereotypical picture of a dotty scientist studying love lives of arcane creatures, to the uncritical acceptance of highly speculative hypotheses as straight fact. As the late Professor Lehrman has pointed out so well in this volume, the offering and receiving of these notions often has to do with the promotion or support of a dearly held prejudgment. The social issues involved are enormously important. Thinking about them should be as informed and free of prejudice as possible.

The readership for which this book is written includes the vast array of psychiatrists, psychiatry residents, clinical psychologists, social workers, medical students, and others for whom the use of animal data to clarify human behaviour is of practical or curious importance. In addition, it may serve to orient the many postgraduate and undergraduate students in psychology and other biological sciences to this important stream of ideas in psychiatry today. Finally, the book is tailored to the presumed tastes and needs of the interested but inexpert general reader. It requires only a passing acquaintance with either field to be understood.

There is a loose grouping of chapters according to their content. At first glance, several of them appear to be rather technical discussions of ethological esoterica. In fact, the research data are exemplary, because the authors address themselves mainly to problems involved in the transfer of ideas from one field to the other. The introduction is written from a psychiatric point of view and, in a cursory review of the literature, shows what has already been done to link the two fields. The bibliographies have been arranged at the end of the volume, in a way which provides a source of easy reference to readings in ethology and its connections with the human behavioural sciences.

The book originated in a seminar at McMaster University, 28-30 September 1970, as the Third Hincks Memorial Lecture. This lectureship was established in memory of Clarence M. Hincks, widely regarded as the father of the Canadian mental health movement. It is co-sponsored by the Ontario Mental Health Foundation and five Ontario medical schools through which it is rotated annually, and has become a major platform for statements on human behaviour. In the autumn of 1969, Professor N.B. Epstein, chairman of the McMaster Department of Psychiatry, polled its members to choose a topic, format, and speaker for the coming lecture. The consensus was that we should use the occasion to explore unfamiliar ground and that the usual academic ritual should be subordinate to the exchange and extension of views – a difficult task, considering the way most meetings happen. The department's dual interest in family therapy and in the use of biological sciences to teach psychiatry biased our choice as the possible and interesting topics were gradually narrowed down and there emerged a design for a working conference on 'The Application of Ethology to Human Growth and Development.' Since the whole purpose was to bring ideas together, we planned to have a number of carefully selected participants engage in an extended and intimate work session as free of performance restraints as possible. Attendance was to be limited, with less formal presentation than actual discussion between the participants. We asked Professor Hinde to deliver the keynote address. He, and each of our first choices of workshop leaders and participants, accepted. Our guest seminarians were told that we did not plan to publish the proceedings, but that the gathering was intended to provide an opportunity for exchange of ideas. The meeting itself began on a Monday afternoon with a screening of several films on animal behaviour, most of them provided by members of the conference faculty who responded to questions after each film. That night the address by Dr Hinde was formally discussed by Dr Kaufman. During the following two days, the time was divided into four workshops: 'Mother/Infant Relations'; 'Organization of Group Patterns'; 'Evolutionary models of Behaviour'; 'Highlights of Problems in the Application of Human Growth and Development.' The meeting was a huge success – sufficiently so that at lunch on Wednesday the participants agreed that contrary to the original plan, the proceedings ought to be published in some form. Thus the eventual shape of the book has been determined by the fact that its authors had to write their contributions after the meeting. Although the general thrust is the same as what occurred there, the chapters differ somewhat from the transcript. Also, the freedom of the conference design resulted in, among other things, some departure from its founding theme. Therefore, the internal organization of the book does not correspond to that originally set for the meeting, and its title reflects the change in focus.

One of the lessons to emerge from the experience of publishing this volume is that although meetings are a long time in the making, books are longer still. For the original success of the former, making it possible for the participants to contribute so effectively, credit and thanks are due to Dr J.R. Evans, Dr N.B. Epstein, Dr J.M. Cleghorn, Dr E.A. Griffin, Mr J.H. Cohen, Miss Elaine Edwards, Mr Rick Cuciurean, and the Ontario Mental Health Foundation chaired by Mr A. Posluns Sr. For such merit as it has, but for none of its flaws, the final preparation of this volume owes a debt to the patient, critical, and skilled assistance of Dr D.S. Bishop, Dr J.M. Cleghorn, Dr B.G. Galef, Dr G. Molnar, Dr S.L. Smith, Dr M. Spinner, Dr N. Spinner, Mrs D. Novak, and Mrs M.J. Rubenstein.

NORMAN F. WHITE

---

† During the preparation of this volume, we were saddened to learn of Dr Lehrman's death on 29 August 1972. He was widely respected and fondly regarded by his associates in a broad and complex field. Also, as might be inferred from his chapter in this book, he was well known for his concern about important social problems. At the Hincks conference itself, his co-participants were treated to a fluent and provocative statement of the kind which, as colleagues, they had come to expect from him. The audience was captivated as he took some of the most difficult questions that had arisen and wove them together, not only dextrously, but apparently extempore. The manuscript which was developed from these remarks appears as Dr Lehrman's very searching and elaborate question in chapter eleven: 'Can Psychiatrists Use Ethology?'

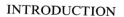

INTRODUCTION

NORMAN F. WHITE

Ethology and Psychiatry

A psychiatrist would be liable to say that the ultimate concern of all biology is man. Some scientists may quarrel with this view, but it is difficult to avoid human possibilities in the work of those who study animal behaviour. Especially is this so, it would appear, in the case of ethologists, whose field of study includes the social aspects of animal life. Hence, the psychiatrist's interest in ethology. Behaviour and all its physical, social, and ancestral origins is what both ethology and psychiatry are about. It has become fashionable, moreover, to see a convergence of the two around an under- standing of the 'real' character of man — which has meant, whatever one makes of the original proposition, looking at man as a species: how he got here, and how well he is doing. Not only do the disciplines share a concern with the way organisms adapt to their milieux, they also see the complex events of such adaptation as a process within which behaviour stems from an interaction between the organism's structure and its setting. From a psychi- atrist's point of view, failure to cope with the environment results in the symptoms which have become his stock-in-trade. For an ethologist, variations in adaptational success are important in determining the very nature of the species. He presumes that present modes of behaviour have come to exist through the rigours of evolution, and attempts to understand the lineage of behaviour patterns in a way that will explain the acts and reactions of modern animals. Although clinicians do not ordinarily think about human dys- function in such phylogenetic terms, this kind of inference does bear some resemblance to what happens in the formulations of dynamic psycho- pathology. Here, a belief in the ontogenetic determinism of disordered behaviour has bred systematic developmental schemata in which explanations of current behaviour can be sought. There is a kinship of both style and content between the two groups of behavioural scientists that, taken beyond mere historical curiosity, requires that we ask, specifically and practically, whether the findings of ethology are applicable to psychiatric questions.

Ethology has been variously described as the biology of behaviour, the comparative study of behaviour, the study of the social behaviour of animals, and the study of animal behaviour in its native setting. Together, these definitions roughly encompass a modern version of this field of study. Its name, however, has had a long history and other meanings. At about the same time that *The Origin of Species* (Darwin, 1859) was published, Geoffroy Saint-Hilaire coined the word 'ethology,' referring to the study of animals in their native habitat. He was unaware of another English usage, persisting until early in this century, which pertained to the science of moral character formation ('the exact science of human nature'; J.S. Mill, 1843). Although the biological sense of the word fell into disuse for some time, the distinction it had originally furnished — between naturalistic biology and what came, about 1900, to be known as 'comparative psychology' — endured. Incorporating the ideas of ecology the term was kept alive by Giard and Wheeler through the latter part of the nineteenth century into the 1920s, then by Lorenz and Tinbergen until after the second world war. Spirited and competitive disputes between psychologists and ethologists have since subsided into a more ecumenical ecology-focused biology of behaviour (Fletcher, 1957; Jaynes, 1969; Lehrman, 1963). Ethology is now generally accepted as referring to the comparative study of behaviour in a natural setting (Eibl-Eibesfeldt and Kramer, 1958; Thorpe, 1956; Tinbergen, 1951).

Instinct versus Learning

The essential orientation of ethology is to the relationship between organisms and their environments. Underlying this approach, however, is a basic question about the origin of behaviour. Are behavioural events preordained ('programmed') by the structure of the organism, and their environmental setting important only as a stage on which they can be played out? Or does the milieu influence the way behaviour occurs, and eventually the nature of the apparatus itself? The recent history of ethology has revolved largely around this question — that is, about 'learning' and its apparent converse, 'instinct.' The problem has been to determine whether certain behaviours are 'acquired' or 'innate.' The interplay of these complementary properties of behavioural development has been a major and sometimes contentious issue between ethologists and psychologists (Beech, 1955; Fletcher, 1957; Hebb, 1953; Lehrman, 1953; Thorpe, 1956). Centuries before the arrival of ethology, it had been appreciated that many animals (including, to some extent, man) have ways of acting and living that are peculiar to themselves and unvarying enough that certain adaptational and behavioural patterns can be regarded as quite stable. Yet it had not been clear whether these behaviours were innate or acquired, and they often seemed to be both. For example, von Pernau had noted, in the early eighteenth century, that some birds had to learn their songs while others sang in a species-characteristic way without ever having heard conspecifics sing. In contrast to many examples of learned behaviour, Spalding showed (1873) that swallows deprived of any opportunity to use their wings could fly as soon as given the chance. Zoologists and people from other disciplines were attracted to the problem, and their work culminated around the end of the nineteenth century in such formal definitions of instinct as that by the psychologist William James. One effect of this interest was to kindle a controversy – innate versus acquired, or instinct versus learning – which has lasted in psychology right up to the current furious wrangle about intelligence and its testing.

Phylogeny

The nature-nurture argument, sometimes tedious and unproductive, has nonetheless increased our understanding of behaviour, because its resolution depends on the idea that there is seldom (if ever) a clear distinction between innate and acquired. Behind this insight is the realization that behaviours, much like fins, flippers, and limbs, evolve. In order to imagine such a process, we require the concept of *phylogeny:* the evolutionary development of types of organisms – the history of divergence from a common stock through the influence of selection. The degrees of 'innateness' and the means by which it is modifiable, are subject to phylogenetic analysis in ways elaborated later in this volume. Hinde (1970), in proposing that we put the innate-acquired controversy finally to rest, has suggested we speak of 'environmentally stable or labile' behaviours. He sees learning expressed in behaviour, and instinct, as different aspects of an interaction between the organism and the environment, and both as being subject to the pressures of selection (Hinde and Tinbergen, 1953). This general view has been latent for some time. Its foundation was laid when Darwin altered the course of all biological thought in his exposition of selective principles. He was evidently quite sensitive to the environment's role in determining the shape of adaptive behaviour, and anticipated the concerns of present-day ethologists in *The Descent of Man* (1871) and *The Expression of Emotion in Man and Animals* (1873). George John Romanes continued this development with his *Mental Evolution in Animals* (1884) and *Mental Evolution in Man* (1889). Thereafter, a succession of thinkers ushered the idea of change by selective adaptation through to this day, though the emphasis was seldom on behaviour.

The brilliant vision of Darwin still required, however, some accompanying operational models before it could be translated into scientific investigation. The key idea was, of course, contained in the long-mislaid thesis of Gregor Mendel. His theory of genetic inheritance provided an intergenerational explanation for the transmission of characteristics. Next, Morgan (1896) wrote about the evolutionary background of the nervous system and, in effect, described the history of the apparatus which mediates the expression of instincts. Then, with his hypothesis that ontogeny recapitulates phylogeny, Haeckel (1910) proposed a way that a condensed version of this history could be seen in the individual organism. When similarities of behaviour systems between species were demonstrated by Heinroth (1910) and Whitman (1919), a kind of behavioural taxonomy could be elaborated from what Darwin had originally proposed.

Analytic examination of the behaviour patterns themselves was begun by William Craig in 1918 when he first distinguished between *appetitive* behaviours and *consummatory* acts. In order to analyse the relation of any such complex activities to their milieu, certain assumptions were necessary. Von Uexküll (1909), for example, posited that the organism responds only to the extent that the environment affects its perceptual apparatus. His *umwelt* concept was useful in showing that this 'perceived' part of its surroundings becomes, as far as the organism is concerned, the whole environment.

Modern Ethology: Terminology

Konrad Lorenz began to bring these ideas together during the 1930s, focusing on a detailed study of innate motor patterns. He described apparently spontaneous acts, the events which triggered them, and the evolution of both of these. This was a phylogenetic analysis which prepared the ground for much of what has become familiar in the field. Niko Tinbergen, at one time Lorenz' student and popularly regarded as a co-founder of ethology, studied extensively the social acts of insects, fish, and birds. These two authors, beginning around 1950, were largely responsible for the first widely circulated ethological writings, and for the modest vogue they acquired. The subject area began to be recognizable (and, one might say, viable) as a discipline with the arrival of a generation of 'ethologists' equipped to establish a critical dialogue with their predecessors (e.g., Lehrman, 1953). Ethology had been reborn. There rapidly developed a special vocabulary which referred to the things ethologists were studying and talking about. To the consternation of its proprietors, some of this new language was reduced to a list of ill-understood catch-words that have too often served to introduce ethology to people in other fields, including psychiatry. There have been easy and misleading equations which Moltz, for example, as long ago as 1936 cautioned against when he distinguished the 'fixed action pattern' from traditional instincts. The ethologists who express concern about the misuse of these words, particularly when confused with vernacular terms, feel that a standardized jargon tends to define ethology somewhat inaccurately. Even though some of the common terms are outdated, familiarity with them is handy for reading in or about the field, because they still appear regularly. That is, for example, one should be aware that *fixed action patterns* (FAP) are stereotyped innately-determined behaviours which occur when *released* by a particular environmental *sign stimulus* which *unlocks* an *innate releasing mechanism* (IRM), and that the *action-specific energy* which propels such behaviour can be depleted by repetition and restored by rest. In the absence of stimuli, it can result in *vacuum activity* and two competing stimuli may be responded to with *displacement behaviour* which ordinarily would be appropriate to a third stimulus. *Ritualization,* we learn, occurs through evolution when a behavioural fragment is retained from a more complex act, taking on a *signalling* function. One of the earliest apparently innate behaviours shown by an infant bird or mammal is *imprinting* — following and forming a bond with an object presented at the right time — and this may be taken to demonstrate the *interlocking* of environmental and innate elements in the expression of instinctive behaviour. The time during which bonding can occur may be regarded as the first *critical period* in development, because before or after a species-constant interval, such a response is difficult or impossible to elicit. This is the classical glossary of ethology. To many, its words have a faintly biblical ring. Their meanings do not represent a coherent theoretical structure but a rather unsystematic collection of things observed and inferred in the formative years of ethological thought.

More recently, ethology has greatly expanded in scope. Its technical language now must accommodate the demands of excursions into phylogeny, linguistics, endocrinology, neurophysiology, and studies of social group interactions. This ever more catholic array of terms indicates the direction and rapidity of the development of ethology over the past two decades (Eibl-Eibesfeldt, 1970; Ewer, 1968; Fox, 1968a; Hess, 1962, 1967; Hinde, 1970; Klopfer, 1967; Mason and Riopelle, 1964). Part of the picture has been a divergence between classical Lorenzian ethology and 'social ethology.' In Crook's (1970a) description of this schism, he points to 'human ethology' as a possible development of the latter. There are several excellent accounts of the evolution of ethology as a discipline and as a science (Barnett, 1963; Beer, 1963; Jaynes, 1969; Tinbergen, 1963). The proselytic fervour of those who hold the ethological point of view is quite compelling. So persuasive have they been, however, in attracting converts from other fields, that it is increasingly evident that ethology is, as much as anything else, an attitude. The eventual absorption of this way of thinking by other, older, and more sovereign disciplines is inevitable. Whether it will retain any independent scientific identity is less certain, but we shall doubtless see the influence of ethology in other subjects, such as psychiatry.

WHITHER PSYCHIATRY?

The recent history of psychiatry has been dominated less by the technology of behaviour control than by flux in its tasks and role in society. Professionally, there has been a diversification which may well have some paradoxical results. All manner of things – criminality, connubial dissatisfaction, senile deterioration, suicide – now come within the purview of behavioural clinicians. These guardians of conventional polity see a wide variety of cases where bad social fit, unfulfilled personal goals, or nuclear angst do not agreeably submit to the Procrustean reductionism of medical diagnosis. Consequently, there has been a proliferation of remedial techniques, due not so much to an improvement of the craft as to a frenetic extension of responsibility. Methods of 'treatment' range from friendly exhortation to cortical extirpation – with stops along the way at reliving primal agonies, token economics, drugs, psychotherapy, and so on.

Methods and Models

However, beneath the fast shuffle of therapeutic chic, one can discern trends in the serious thinking of clinical behavioural scientists. Along with a change in the nature of the problems he considers, the psychiatrist has also changed his approach to them. The most conspicuous thrust of the past three decades has been an inclination to look more outside the person to explain his distress or dysfunction. In dynamic psychiatry, for example, the reorientation of psychoanalytic thought to the 'adaptive' position of so-called 'ego psychology' was a concession to the pressure of clinicians and theoreticians who could no longer ignore the interplay of psychic and environmental forces. The ecological spin-off from this development has resulted in transcultural psychiatry, group therapy techniques, family psychiatry, and community psychiatry. There has been increasing interest in the interactions of individuals, and in the things that happen between people and their total adaptation-demanding envelope. Publicly less dramatic, but hardly less important, has been the steady progress of biological psychiatry – that is, in the effort to uncover intra-organismic determinants in the pathology of behaviour and experience. Least apparent of all, because it verges on being a professional secret, is the growing difference between these approaches. There was, at one time, a clear schism between the socio-therapeutic psychiatrists and their biologic counterparts. The lingo of this conflict labelled the two camps 'dynamic' and 'organic.' By dint of great effort and conviction, the gap seemed to have been quite effectively bridged. It now threatens to open once more, because the public purser is increasingly reluctant to support both ends of the clinical endeavour. Some special augury would be required to foretell exactly how this rupture might occur, but certain general developments are likely. The casualties of social misadventure, whose rescue, relief, or salvage do not require the application of medical expertise, will probably become the province of some other social aid apparatus. What remains 'in' psychiatry, at least at a clinical level, will be more definitely biological in character, and both the activities and the composition of training programmes will reflect this. However, despite any such shift in clinical emphasis, the connections between social phenomena and organismic functions cannot but continue to be very important. The special task of academic psychiatry will be to link and combine the sub-specialty methods of looking at problems. The psychiatric theoretician will be concerned with how we unite the insights of the behavioural and the social sciences. Descriptions of neuronal microfunctions and epidemiological data alone, or together, are not much help to us. To be useful, their organization into working systems must be understood. The detail and subtlety of soma and society are unquestionably the foundation of any serious approach to human behaviour, but it is the macrophenomena which are psychiatry's legitimate and special object of study.

The breadth of an enterprise which attempts a synthetic explanation of so many things is intimidating. None of the major theoretical formulations in the sacrament of psychiatry has proven sufficient by itself and, moreover, it appears that the day of the big theory is gone. The all-encompassing elegance of the psychoanalytic adventure which had such an effect on Western culture is now often viewed by psychiatry students with such indifference that former critics of the theory find themselves, out of scholarly conscience, becoming apologists for it. Systems theory has been an attempt, using a kind of conceptual diplomacy, to achieve broad theoretical assemblage but, at the cost of becoming a non-theory, has succeeded largely in demonstrating the extreme difficulty of doing so. In effect, by setting out a framework within which all theories are compatible and to which the contribution of each can be made without doing too much violence to its own logic, it suggests that there really cannot be a comprehensive theory of human existence. We ought to learn from this to seek theories and conceptual models applicable to only limited areas of behaviour and experience. Students, it follows, should be taught that theoretical models be judged according to their utility, not their 'truth,' and should learn the hazards of mistaking a conceptual tool for insight into the way things really are.

Role

For the present, there is a pragmatic problem, with ingredients that are many and complex. This bears directly on the psychiatrist's role. He must blend the approximate with the shopworn and the metaphorical to come up with precision enough for his conscience – and lay on with hands to fill the gaps. Looking at ordinary behaviour, we know it to be affected by so many things that it is practically unclassifiable. 'Abnormal behaviour,' aside from the problem of its definition, is scarcely less difficult to catalogue. But even with improvements in labelling, psychiatrists are less and less satisfied with cramming multiplex human distress into traditional medical nosologies. They know that specific treatments for specific maladies are the exception. For the rest, a wise and creative clinician avoids random groping for nostra by imposing method on his improvisation. The work is less art than craft. When it is enlightened improvisation, applying a wide repertoire of techniques and devices to the ameliorative tasks of its practitioners, the sobriquet 'eclectic' becomes a compliment. But then role becomes a problem of identity. Who is this clinical jack-of-all-trades? What of these means and their divers origins, and can we tell which of them are really 'psychiatric'? Psychiatry has been, to some degree, a non-discipline. Scratch any psychiatric puzzle and a question appears couched in the language of physiology, sociology, or semantics. Send a student of psychiatry to the source material of a clinical formulation and he will return with the work of an anatomist, a philosopher, or a pharmacologist. When psychiatrists have worn the guise and spoken the tongue of other disciplines it has always been with a faint and uncomfortable aura of imposture. However, clinical problem-solving does require a combination of models and tools that rises above mere dilettantism. Perhaps it is just this synthetic task which is uniquely psychiatric.

THE PROBLEM OF CLINICAL THEORY

Ethology has been commended as a branch of biology which has resisted the move of its parent psychological discipline toward the respectability of clean, well-counted laboratory experimentation. While modern ethologists certainly know and use sophisticated research design, they retain their original bias that behaviour out of its natural setting is fundamentally different from that which occurs in the situation for which selection has adapted it. They have not regarded the multiplicity of environmental factors as contaminants, but as relevant parts of an interactive process, feeling that something important would be lost in an exclusively atomistic search for behaviour sources. Through their effort, the point has been made that a naturalistic approach is scientifically legitimate. This is reminiscent of respectability problems psychiatry has had in its own medical milieu. Mensural zeal has often led to the collection of very hard data based on very soft concepts. It is obvious that there are important questions which psychiatry cannot yet answer by careful measuring in clean experimental situations. It is no longer considered nihilistic to seek an understanding of psychological events outside of Baconian data-gathering. There is clearly something more to empiricism than arithmetic. Strangely, it is not sufficiently appreciated that this caveat should also extend to the examination of clinical phenomena. Here too, in what is necessarily the antithesis of the uncontaminated experimental situation, it is important that there is a place for a naturalistic approach which, though rigorous, does not conform to the strictures of conventional research design.

Faced with a scramble of interrelated phenomena, some important and some not, clinicians try to winnow out those items to which they should direct their remedial attention. They make subtle and arbitrary judgments that simplify their field of operation and impose some conceptual order upon it — and, truth be told, they do it with less than uniform success. Such attempts at conceptual precision co-exist with their necessary but sometimes reluctant awareness that treatment is an essentially human process. That is, the treatment situation resists our efforts to simplify it, and is thus unavoidably 'contaminated.' Even in the relatively few psychiatric conditions for which specific treatments can be prescribed with clear-cut indications, good clinical teaching demands that other things not be ignored. For example, when lithium carbonate is administered to govern the racing thoughts of a manic state, it is often supplemented by another agent given for the control of hyperkinesis and, further, both are likely to be rendered more effective if some attention is paid to the patient's family and to the immediate stresses in his life. Electroplexy for some affective disorders, major tranquillizers for the schizophreniform cognitive disturbances, and disulphiram to interrupt the pathological intake of alcohol are similarly 'specific,' but seldom can be expected to take care of the whole picture. Ordinarily, their use is part of a broader approach and is considered with a view to the vast collection of yearning, fright and social exigency making up each patient's life.

Thus the métier of the psychiatrist is inventive — and so often is the invention intuitive that a major theme in modern psychiatric training is the use of 'feelings' in clinical decision-making. In spite of a rapidly increasing fund of data and documented behavioural insights, it will always be intrinsically psychiatric to improvise in advance of the data in order to understand an individual human situation. This is commonly supposed to be the clinical art, about which so much impassicned nonsense has been written. The choice has seemed to be between the logical unaccountability of the artist and the search for the one more biochemical connection, slightly improved nosology, or subtle new conditioning schedule which will take us out of this imprecision. Obviously, even though their flaws are easy to caricature, neither stance is wholly wrong. The trouble with an artistic approach is that the logical structure it operates within is likely to be the private and culture-bound aesthetic of the individual clinician. This is at least human, its advocates say, and better than the mechanistic and ceremonial illusions of the science cult. Clinical theory, if it is not to founder on the rhetoric that stretches between crisp rigour and latter-day humanism, needs a conceptual framework that will accommodate quite different kinds of ideas. Enter ethology.

THE AFFINITY

Does ethology really have enough in common with psychiatry that any natural relation can be said to exist between their students? Perhaps so. Although ethology can appear to be a fairly consistent set of theoretical notions, it utilizes, like psychiatry, the tools of several other disciplines. Ethology, again like psychiatry, has learnt to develop and re-vamp techniques for its own purposes. Each field is a mosaic of such specialties as neurophysiology, developmental psychology, communications theory, and genetics. They are hybrid in origin and broad in their points of view. It is an ethological truism that no student of the native behaviour of an animal can understand his subject if he does not account for its developmental history, the behavioural traditions in which this development occurs, the character of the environment as experienced by the animal, the effects of individual behaviours on each other, the neurophysiological apparatus emitting such behaviours, and the interactions between each and all these things. Except that it would be unreasonably ambitious, the same statement could be made about a psychiatrist. Only lately, but nonetheless quite definitely, can psychiatry be said to aspire to the breadth of synthesis on which the existence of ethology has depended from its beginnings. Recognizably ethological writings have been available for about fifty years — say, since Heinroth. For about half that time ethology has been a labelled discipline. In spite of this, it has not even become one of a series of intellectual fashions in psychiatry, much less seriously adopted. The scattered references and loose allusions to contributions ethology might make have never developed into a rapprochement which explored the implications of such a partnership. It has perhaps taken this long for psychiatry to conclude its exclusive dependence on 'psychopathology' to explain behavioural dysfunction. If there is a special affinity between ethology and psychiatry it is probably in the *general* analysis of behaviour. It is here that psychiatry may benefit most. Yet beyond the ethologist's insistence that behaviour be viewed as part of an ontological and phyletic process in a richly detailed environment, the query stands: How do we use animals to understand people?

To the Human Species

Animal studies have puzzled and fascinated psychiatrists for a long time. During the ebb and flow of arguments about their general relevance, there has been a more-or-less constant interest in the syndromes, learning behaviours, and stress responses observable in lesser creatures. Critics of, for example, 'rat psychology' have questioned whether such simulations permit any useful inference to the human case, rejecting species analogism as an alternative to the subjectivist study of mental phenomena. Behaviourism, withal, could hardly have become established but for a heavy reliance on animal experimentation, and it still plays an important role. In modern psychiatry, bioassay pharmacology has been combined with this accumulated knowledge of animal behaviour to develop and refine drug treatments. Emphasis on the biochemical and physiological origins of mental disorder has led to experiments where parts of the brain have been stimulated or removed − in animals, of course. It is only recently that any micro-electrode implantation has been attempted in the human species, and the examination of extirpation sequelae in people is confined to 'natural experiments' that result from accidents, surgery, or intracranial disease. Some findings from animal work in this area have had broad implications for human neurophysiology, notably in the study of mid-brain functions (Drewe et al., 1970; MacLean, 1972). Journals regularly publish reviews of animal research germane to human psychology (Mason and Riopelle, 1964; Wood-Gush, 1963) against a background of receding doubt regarding the legitimacy of inferences taken from such studies. As Tiger (1969) has said, it 'may be astonishing to future historians that it was doubted that there were important behaviour affinities.' In an earlier review of the significance of these studies, Hebb and Thompson (1954) assure us that their relevance is perfectly clear, but insist that man must still be thought of as quite distinct. Considering the amount of work done, and an apparently widespread faith in its importance, the results of animal research have been peculiarly disappointing. Information obtained from studies of experimental neurosis has yet to show us the etiology or treatment of a single major psychiatric malady. In the area of human development, where the application of animal data has been especially attractive, Ambrose (1968) has noted the unfulfilled early promise of animal learning studies.

Psychiatric training programmes continue to include this material in their 'basic sciences.' However, students often ask, 'What does this animal work have to do with what I want to learn about treating people?' The answer to this is by no means clear, and it points out some uncertainty as to how, in fact, such data ought to be applied to clinical theory. Reasoning by crude analogy, inference is direct and simple: what we see in animals is an attenuated or parallel version of what occurs in humans. It is all the more tempting to think in this fashion because there is an impressive tradition of physiological research which appears to bear out its validity. However, few researchers in psychiatry would doubt that this way of thinking breaks down for the events of the mind. It is not, for these purposes, even necessary to be clear about what the mind is. It could, indeed, be defined as that thing influencing human behaviour which cannot ordinarily be considered to be present in other species. Thus, we are liable to be misled when seeking in animals phenomena which can be treated as simple analogues of the human case. The difficulty is compounded by the conventional and implicit assumption in psychiatry that causes are to be found in lesions. In contradistinction to process, a lesion can be located – if not anatomically, then at least functionally. Ergo, isolated workings in parts of the nervous apparatus of other species have seemed to be a reasonable thing to look at in order to understand human distress and dysfunction – themselves explicable by finding out more about isolated events in our own brains. It turns out, of course, not to be so. In fact, it appears that the problem of knowing how to use animal research data is part of a problem of knowing how to use any data. Therefore, it may be that learning how to apply the findings of animal research will illuminate the psychiatrist's more general question about which elements of human experience and behaviour he selects for study.

Man differs from other species (though perhaps only in degree) in that social structures of his own device alter and steer his actions. Socially affected behaviours quickly become 'traditional' and, in turn, modify their own social context. There is a spiral of response-effect-response that takes us, phenomenologically, further and further away from the physical biological bases of our acts. We can thus expect whatever physical biological laws operate in behaviour to be buried beneath layers of socio-interactional complexities. Behaviour genetics and its epidemiological cousin, population genetics, have been widely used in psychiatry to study mental illness. The dilemma has been to determine which of the things we observe should be regarded as 'physical' in origin, and which to think of in another way. In some cases, it could be quite incorrect to view a piece of behaviour as having 'evolved' genetically — that is, viewing it as a result of a physical property to which a phylogenetic string is attached. Ethology may be able to show psychiatrists to which elements of behaviour they ought to apply the special logic of phylogeny. Less obviously, it may also provide a conceptual model for the evolution of social behaviours. This is clinically important. It would probably be easier to decide what heritable factors should be sought in 'depression,' for example, if the remote adaptive utility of responses resembling or contributing to a 'pathological' pattern in the syndrome were understood. In another example, 'schizophrenia' has long posed a nosological and descriptive problem. It has been clear for some time that certain aspects of this disease (or family of disorders) may be transmitted from one generation to another. We would be better able to decide which and how if we understood better which elements of behaviour patterns are more environmentally labile than others, and what may be the kinds of principles or laws governing their formation, modification, and descent.

Different kinds of information can be applied from animal research to psychiatry, and there are different ways this can be done. One may distinguish three *orders of complexity* in the data and concepts which make up that part of ethological thinking which is of interest to psychiatry: *(a) physiological*, anatomical, and biochemical; *(b) micro-organizational*, individual behaviour; *(c) macro-organizational*, in social behaviours. Each of them has something to offer the student of human behaviour, for whom there are three *types of utilization*: (i) *direct transposition*; (ii) the *imposition of models*; (iii) the *application of the techniques* used by ethologists. The

	Utilization		
Complexity	*direct transposition*	*imposition of models*	*application of the techniques*
Physiological		XXXXXXXXXXXXXXXXXX XXXXXXXXXXXXXXXXXXX	
Micro-organizational		XXXXXXXXXXXXXXXXXXXXXX XXXXXXXXXXXXXXXXXXXXXX	
Macro-organizational		XXXXXXXXXXXXXXXXXXX XXXXXXXXXXXXXXXXX	

findings, of Hydén and Reisen (not ethologists) about the physical consequences of early developmental events are widely accepted to be directly translatable to the human case. On the other hand, the formulations of Papez, MacLean, and Olds regarding the functions of the limbic system and related structures have greatly influenced psychiatric thinking, but more as models within which a variety of neuro-behavioural data may be understood. The human application of methods (microelectrodes, etc.) to explore these phenomena has been attempted by Heath and some others. Similarly, examples of individual and social behavioural phenomena may be fitted into the remainder of this conceptual grid. All types of utilization are legitimate, with the caveat that it should be quite clear exactly how transposition to the human case is being effected. So far, the particular relevance of ethology to psychiatry seems to have fallen mainly into the areas of models and methods to explain and explore individual and social behaviour. Finally, as it emphasizes a comparative approach to analysis, ethology can be expected to add yet another dimension to the examination of behavioural problems.

THE LITERATURE

Considering the quantity of literature addressed to the significance of animal studies to human behaviour, there has been relatively little specific reference to ethology in psychiatric publications. This review culls much of what has appeared and is an attempt to provide, in addition to its annotated citations, some indication of themes and trends. The translation of ethological concepts into psychiatric terms has ranged from broad suggestions about how all psychiatry can be seen within an ethological perspective to isolated explanations of particular psychiatric phenomena that have seemed to resemble things reported by students of animal behaviour. Most have concentrated on optimistic proposals for the direct application of data to explain symptoms ('displacement activity' has been especially popular), to open up the mysteries of early development ('imprinting'), or to provide a biological basis for aggression-related behaviour. Referring to arguments about the evolution of incest taboos, Slater (1968) expresses concern about the confusion of homology and analogy in the transfer of models from animal to man. Several suggestions for the use of ethological techniques, such as the 'ethogram,' have been made, but the logical nature of their connection is seldom clarified. Much of the material in this volume bears directly on this issue.

Zegans (1967) has said that in addition to enriching the psychiatric vocabulary with their terms, we owe it to the ethologists that 'even a school child knows that Mary's little lamb did not follow her out of trusting affection but due to a chance imprinting at a critical period.' Kraus (1970) describes evolutionary biology as an 'enigmatic' field offering psychiatry new insights into the human condition. Writing from a pediatric point of view, Ambrose (1968) and Grant (1965) have reviewed the application of the ethological method to psychiatric situations. Ethological propositions, however, have not been accepted uncritically. Birch (1961), particularly doubtful about the application of 'instinct,' stressed the importance of 'continuous reorganization and reintegration' in human behaviour, and warned that the quest for dramatic analogies – particularly to support psychodynamic hypotheses – may be mistaken. While allowing that the application of concepts from one branch of study to another may lead to 'spectacular' advances, Beer (1968) cautions psychoanalysts against a too hasty adoption of some of the ethological notions to which they have been most attracted. Kramer (1968), similarly wary of overinterpretation, nonetheless states that 'activity patterns and the underlying instinctual internal driving factors' are relevant for an understanding of the biology and development of man. Also, ethological findings have been used in a biological examination of the economic and structural hypotheses in psychoanalytic metapsychology (Fletcher, 1957; Kaufman, 1960a; Moses, 1968a; Ostow, 1959, 1960).

The ultimately ambitious application of ethology to psychopathology is Lorenz' (1970) phylogenetic analysis of the imminent destruction of our culture due to a 'mass neurosis,' a situation he has already (1963) said will not be helped by conventional education. In an exchange with Schmidbauer (1971), the same author (1971) defends the case for an examination of large social problems by human ethology. Tinbergen (1968) has said that we can 'go down with some dignity' meeting nature scientifically. There has been some question about the utility of such propositions. Hess (1970), more cautious and closer to the data, does see value in the study of man's 'genetically programmed behaviour.' Yet from beneath a subtitle which says that basing human behaviour on instincts violates 'the findings of developmental biopsychology,' Eisenberg (1972) states that man is his 'own chief product' and takes psychiatric umbrage at the overstatements of ethological popularizers.

There are several areas of special interest to the psychiatrist in which links have been suggested with ethology. In the following sections, where such reference is described, it is interesting to note the contrast between an emphasis on laboratory-derived findings and the basic ethological position regarding 'naturalistic' data. Furthermore, whatever the source of the data, their interpretation is guided by no obvious constant rationale.

Growth and Development

One of the first writers to make a specific connection between ethology and psychiatry was John Bowlby (1951, 1957, 1958, 1960). His observations on the enduring consequences of maternal deprivation and the debate engendered by his numerous publications have led to a great deal of research on the psychophysiological factors which determine healthy development in its earliest stages (Ainsworth, 1962; Bridger, 1962; Bronfenbrenner, 1968; Casler, 1961; O'Connor, 1968; Rutter, 1972; Schur, 1960, 1961; Yarrow,

1965). Extensive work by Harlow (1959, 1962, 1963, 1965) on the development of affectional systems in rhesus monkeys, and his demonstration of the intergenerational effects of deprivation have had a significant influence on psychiatric thinking in this area. The primary social bond (Freedman et al., 1961; Schneirla et al., 1961; Scott, 1962, 1963) has become a major focus of attention and its parental aspects were the subject of an extensive review by Kaufman (1970). Hinde, in a series of reports (1962, 1967a, 1969, 1970a, 1971), has demonstrated variations and intricacies of the mother-infant dyad and its disruption. The natural history of the maternal contribution to this relationship and its humoral component have been described in the rat by Rosenblatt (1969). Fear, as portrayed in behavioural patterns by Bronson (1968), develops in stages that show significant inter-species similarities, and Freedman (1965) makes somewhat the same point. The obvious resemblance of imprinting (Hess, 1959) and critical periods to the sequential schemata of Freud, Erikson, and Piaget has, as might have been expected, provoked some comment (Ambrose, 1963; Bowlby, 1958; Brody and Axelrad, 1966; Bronson, 1962, 1965; Freedman, 1968; Gray, 1958; Hinde, 1962; Kaufman, 1960; Sluckin, 1964; Taketomo, 1968; Vaughan, 1966).

Drives, needs, and instincts are central to the explanations or problems of any developmental theory, and are considered from a comparative point of view by Barnett (1961) and Kaufman (1960a). Hinde's formulations on drives (1959), suggesting that over-simplified concepts may hinder behavioural analysis, have clarified many of these questions. Somewhat broader syntheses of an ethological approach to the junior years have been offered by Ambrose (1968), Barnett (1962), and Grant (1965). Conceptual links between ethology and the study of both early and later development are detailed in articles by Caldwell (1968), Eibl-Eibesfeldt (1967), Hess (1970), Mason (1968), and Tobach and Schneirla (1968). The development implications of primate research, in particular, have been comprehensively outlined by Jensen and Bobbitt (1968).

Patterns of Social Behaviour

In a recent review of infrahuman social behaviour, Scott (1968) asserts that the basic biosocial nature of man 'defines the limits of satisfactory adaptation to cultural variation.' The dynamics of groups and the behaviour of individuals in groups would seem to be one of the most obvious topics in psychiatry to be examined from an ethological point of view (Kraus, 1970). Contributions in this area, while interesting, remain scant (Kummer, 1971; Morton, 1972). Special situations, such as nursery schools (Blurton-Jones, 1967; Zegans, 1967), normal children (Hutt et al., 1963), state hospital populations (Esser, 1965) and small towns (Barker, 1968) have been analysed using techniques reminiscent of field studies reported by ethologists. The concept of territoriality, extensively reviewed by Carpenter (1964) and Hediger (1961) is applied (Coleman, 1968; Hall, 1959, 1966; Horowitz, 1968), along with dominance (Esser et al., 1965; Price, 1967), to psychiatric patients and psychopathology. Roth (1971) has studied the establishment of homosexual 'territories' in a prison population. The use of space by animals and man received extensive treatment in a recent symposium (Esser, 1971). Davis (1962), examining 'gang' phenomena from a phylogenetic position, suggests ecological solutions to their aggressive consequences. Considered in an adaptive context, play activities appear to have a number of important functions across many species, including *Homo sapiens* (Dolhinow, 1971; Eibl-Eibesfeldt, 1970; Loizos, 1967; Suomi and Harlow, 1971). Some patterns of play and adult gregarious activity shared by humans and other vertebrates are considered by Graham (1964) to be potentially dangerous atavisms when occurring in civilized behaviour. Drawing several parallels between psychodynamic concepts, such as 'identification' and 'superego,' Imanishi (1965) has examined the developmental basis of social structures in wild Japanese monkeys in rather human terms. Tiger and Fox (1966) have proposed in general terms that if social data were to be collected in ways that could be analysed by ethological methods, we could achieve a beneficial marriage of sociology and ethology for the better understanding of human social behaviour.

Aggression

The huge importance of aggression as a social and clinical problem makes it hardly surprising that ethological formulations in the area have stimulated both research and speculation. Price (1969) has extrapolated to the human case a variety of ways in which conspecifics avoid destructive violence by the use of signals and ritualized appeasement manoeuvres. Further, it has been suggested that the origins of the aggressive impulse in territorial or hierarchical conflict may have some analogues in human behaviour (Barnett, 1964; Kraus, 1970). Intriguing as a possible confirmation of current family and social theories, where the affectional sins of parents visit upon their children in the form of anti-social behaviour, maternally inadequate rhesus mothers can be shown to produce hyperaggressive offspring (Arling and Harlow, 1967). The scientific literature on the biology of aggression has expanded rapidly, with a number of reviews appearing (Berkowitz, 1962; Carthy and Ebling, 1964; Clemente and Lindsley, 1967; Daniels et al., 1970; Garrattini and Sigg, 1969; Montagu, 1968; Scott, 1958, 1962a; Storr, 1968).

Tinbergen, who did some of the earlier work in this area, has suggested broader implications for politics and education (1968). Criticized by Montagu (1968) and others as overgeneralized, the popular press has had historical accounts, such as those of Lorenz (1963) and Ardrey (1961, 1966), of man's aggressive behaviour. Specifically, Hinde (1967) challenges Lorenz' insistence on the spontaneity and unmodifiability of aggressiveness. He (Lorenz, 1970) has replied to some of this criticism in a detailed exegesis of the generation gap and its attendant enmities. In an attempt to clarify the concept of 'aggression' itself, Pivnicki (1970) contends that the most misleading feature of ethology is its anthropomorphism, and seems to regret the 'weakness' that psychiatrists have toward ethology. Much of this material is brought together in digestible form in review articles by Fox (1968) and Scott (1970).

Communication

We have seen a number of attempts in psychiatry to catalogue and explain human non-verbal communications both in dyads and in small groups (Bird-whistell, 1959; Ruesch, 1953; Scheflen, 1963). Cross-culturally, Hewes (1957) refers to the 'anthropology of posture.' Eibl-Eibesfeldt (1970), in speaking about 'the ethology of man,' challenges the view that this is learned and socially determined behaviour by confirming the work of many ethologists who have shown striking cross-cultural similarities of emotional expression. The relations between animal and human communication, and the likelihood of general principles applicable to both, have a long history of comment through Haldane (1953, 1955), Hockett (1960), Sebeok (1965), and Bastian (1965). Altmann (1967) has brought together the work of authors from several related fields in a cross-species analysis of the basic nature of social communication. Grant (1965a, 1968), studying social structure in groups of patients and normals, produced physiognomic and gestural descriptions which highlighted their 'essential similarity' of signalling and mood behaviour. This resembles animal work on 'facial' expression which has made it graphically clear that musculo-skeletal and autonomic concomitants in combined states of fear, arousal and other 'emotional' states result in postures which closely resemble none of those resulting from these states alone (Kuhme, 1963; Leyhausen, 1956; Lorenz, 1963). Here is a model which suggests something different from a contemporary psychiatric belief, in spite of difficulty in establishing clear physiological distinctions, that each form of emotional expression must have a corresponding biologic affect state underlying it. This expression (Andrew, 1963; Brown, 1967) and language (Lancaster, 1966) have been traced phylogenetically to primate responses. Zegans (1967) has suggested that problems in perceiving social cues, understandable in ethological terms, may be implicated in paranoid states.

Sexuality

The intricacies of human sexual behaviour, according to Eibl-Eibesfeldt (1970), can be regarded as a complicated system of ritualized signals, the original forms of which led adaptively to species-preserving procreation. The aesthetics of sexuality, which have occupied so much time and attention through man's history, appear to be connected with an array of sexual releasers similar to those seen in primates (Crook and Gartlan, 1966; Wickler, 1967). The cross-cultural prevalence of genital displays has suggested human behavioural vestiges of territorial defence and masculine announcement (Eibl-Eibesfeldt, 1970; Hewes, 1957). Kortmulder (1968) has developed an ethological theory to explain the incest taboo and exogamy.

Sexual inversion in animals has been examined by Hinde (1962a), who proposes that some cases of aberrant sexual activity can be understood as 'behaviour of lower priority appearing when patterns of higher priority are temporarily impossible. Sexual patterns normally characteristic of the other sex may also appear in the presence of those external stimuli which elicit them from the sex in which they normally occur. Inversion of sexual arousal in either sex involves an increased tendency to show both male and female patterns, though the male patterns normally have a higher priority in males and vice versa.' The dual potentiality implied by this view is consistent with recent work in humans (Diamond, 1965; Hampson, 1961; Money, 1965).

Neurosis

Although cautioning against a simple comparison of pathological behaviour in animals and man, Hinde (1962a) has suggested that neurotic behaviour can usefully be studied in animals. He feels that the variety of animal responses to conflict situations, including inhibition, displacement, regression, and immobility 'may influence the complexity of the explanations given for similar cases in man.' In discussing the way these responses become habitually a part of the behavioural repertoire, he stresses the importance of 'sensitive periods' and the divers ways in which early experience can influence later behaviour. Avoidance, stereotypy and superstitious behaviour are examples where such inference may be employed. In contrast to other authors who have said that the absence of abstract thought in animals disqualifies data on their pathological behaviour from application to man, he makes the interesting point that 'man's greater use of conceptual thought often permits more tenuous connections between conflict and symptoms than ever occur in animals.'

Depressions, anxiety and irritability, according to Price (1967) may be seen as 'emotional concomitants of behaviour patterns which are necessary for the maintenance of dominance hierarchies in social groups.' This thesis, in its position that 'depression' helps its bearer to adjust to a lower hierarchical position is consistent with the 'giving-up' (Schmale, 1964) and hibernation (Frank, 1954) theories of depression. Elsewhere, he suggests that human neurotic reaction has evolved as the yielding component of ritual agonistic behaviour (Price, 1969).

Seeking an animal model for depression, several investigators have examined the effects of disrupting the mother/infant bond (Harlow, 1962; Hinde, 1971; Jensen, 1962; Kaufman, 1967, 1967a, 1969; Rosenblum and Kaufman, 1968; Seay, 1962, 1965; Spencer-Booth, 1965). This approach comes from the notion that object-loss and/or deprivation is the origin of the depressive affect or state, and is closely related to the work of Bowlby (1960a) and Spitz (1946) with human infants. By introducing total isolation, peer separation, and physical confinement, Harlow's group has elaborated somewhat on the basic bond/separation paradigm, and has attempted to produce stable depressive states in which a number of social and biological variables can be manipulated (Griffin and Harlow, 1966; Harlow, 1970, 1970a; Harlow, Dodsworth, and Harlow, 1965; Harlow and Suomi, 1971; McKinney, 1971; Suomi, 1972; Suomi, Harlow, and Domek, 1970). In a review of the evidence provided by animal models, McKinney and Bunney (1969) stress the conceptual utility of a 'comparative' approach for the investigation of the enormous clinical problem of depression.

From a 'biodynamic' viewpoint, Masserman (1968) scans the whole range of comparative behavioural research for data relevant to 'normal' and 'abnormal' behaviour, and therapy. In psychosomatics, Engel (1969) has reported a particular type of life situation associated with ulcerative colitis in both gibbon and man, and a connection between displacement behaviour and psychosomatic disorder has been considered (Barnett, 1955). Demaret (1971) essays an explanation of anorexia nervosa in which he claims it has a well-defined biological basis in the survival value of the anorectic's pregnancy avoidance and seemingly paradoxical love of children. He also gives probably the only ethological description of the electral scenario. Assessing phobias, Marks (1969) stresses the phylogenesis of prepotent fear-stimuli, and cites the existence of responses in animals and infants which suggest the 'innate origin' of certain aetiological elements, but emphasizes the primary importance of individual experience.

Kramer (1968) directly addresses the question as to whether *fixed motor patterns* play a role in mental illness. Impulse disorders, tantrums, and moods have been approached rather tentatively in a search for animal equivalents. Tics, and the choreography of social mannerism in such details as tie-straightening and hair-patting, have been equated with *displacement activities* (Eibl-Eibesfeldt, 1970). Similarly, *conflict behaviour* and *intention movements* have been proposed as paradigms for the understanding of neurotic disorders (Grant, 1965; Hess, 1967; Kaufman, 1960; Lorenz, 1957). Bringing together observations on imprinting and the experimental data of classical and operant conditioning, Mitchell (1969) suggests clinical analogies and refers to Menacker's (1956) comments on innate animal behaviours and 'moral masochism' to help in understanding 'the at-one-time adaptive value' of self-defeating and painful behaviour.

Evolution

Through a number of well-known writings, Lorenz has outlined the arguments for behavioural evolution (1952, 1958, 1965). Moses (1968, 1968a) reviews very broadly the humanistic and psychoanalytic import of the evolutionary point of view. Bridger (1962) has pointed out that 'plasticity in all aspects of behaviour increases as one ascends the ladder of phylogenetic development. In order to understand the mechanisms underlying motivated, or goal-directed, behaviour, one should look at the adaptive potential and capacity of the species that governs all forms of its behaviour. To understand [man's] maternal, reproductive, food-getting behaviour one should look for the mechanisms underlying all his adaptive behaviour.'

In the context of human stress biology, Hamburg (1962) remarks that man is best understood in terms of 'how he came to be that way,' and has reviewed the primate evidence for the evolution of emotional responses (1968a). Hamburg (1968) also has made a compelling case for the selective advantage of collective coping strategies in social groups, and has described how such emotional responses facilitate their formation. Useful guidance, he suggests, may be found in the principle that 'individuals seek and find gratifying those situations that have become highly advantageous in survival of the species.' The evolution of hominid behaviour and society has been reviewed several times (Campbell, 1966; Crook, 1970; Fox, 1967; Pfeiffer, 1970; Reynolds, 1966; Rae and Simpson, 1958; Russell and Russell, 1961; Simpson, 1966). Specifically, the evolution of the human family has been proposed in an extended primatological argument which focuses on incest prohibition (Imanishi, 1965a).

The contributions of evolutionary theory and behaviour genetics to psychiatry were surveyed by Brosin (1960), who invoked ethological principles to look at infant behaviour, clinical pragmatics, and pathogenesis. The ontogenetic and phylogenetic development of human dreaming and the REM cycle as described by Roffwarg et al. (1966) and Snyder (1966) touch on what may be the rhythmic elements in human patterns of adaptation. In the most recent of a series of somewhat speculative popular works, Morris (1967,

1969, 1971) elaborates on the evolution and social use of human patterns of physical contact. Barnett (1968) has suggested that we examine the divers phenomena involved in 'teaching' from an ontogentic and from a phylogenetic point of view.

APPLICATIONS

The central theme of ethology since its beginning has sounded an emphasis on the study of animals in their native habitat. Ethologists have recognized that animals in captivity exhibit behaviour peculiar to their special environment. This setting-stereotypy applies also to humans and has important implications for psychiatrists who practise amidst the trappings of an elaborately institutionalized profession. Zegans (1967) has said, 'ethology may make its most important contribution to the study of man by facilitating the accurate and rich description of how people communicate motivational and affective messages to one another in a natural rather than experimental setting.' For 'experimental' read 'office,' and the point is quite clear. Other aspects of special adaptation, such as to the urban environment, have attracted the use of ecological descriptive techniques (Barker, 1968), but to date no serious transfer of models. In these, the potential exists for the clinician to grasp something in the meaning of behaviour beyond the parochial conceit of an anthropomorphic analysis.

Of the major questions which vex theoretical biology, two at least are of immediate interest to a psychiatrist: what is learning? and why does man behave in an apparently non-random way? We begin with the general premise that life is a process of interaction with an environment, during which the organism undergoes some degree of alteration. When this is manifest behaviourally we may refer to 'learning' as having occurred. What is to be altered, the way in which it is altered, and the results of the alteration are, of course, dependent partly on the beginning constitution of the organism. Some alterations are obviously a product of the organism-environment interaction, and since this depends on the state of the organism it follows that these changes are at least partly determined by others that have preceded them. If there were properties of the organism which only became evident some time after its origin, then the course of the interaction would be very much determined by these emergent properties. If, further, they were to emerge in a constant order we would regard the 'development' of the organism as taking place according to a schedule or programme. Similarly, we find that properties are 'expressed' or become manifest under certain regular circumstances, suggesting that some organismic sensitivity to the environment is also programmed. Therefore, 'learning,' whether or not mediated by conscious events, is one aspect of an organism-environment interaction and is dependent upon both aspects of it. Neither the organism nor the environment is entirely unchanged in the process, especially that part of the environment which consists of other organisms. To attribute any behaviour (i.e., any particular interactional event) solely to 'learned' phenomena withour reference to both the original and developed state of the organism is consequently untenable.

There remain elements of 'spontaneity' in behaviour for which this model cannot be expected to account, somewhere within the conflicts between 'mechanism' and 'vitalism,' or 'determinism' and 'free will' — and beyond the uncompromising shallowness of the Skinnerian dialectic. The relevance of these biological questions to the practical behavioural sciences has, in any case, less to do with the ultimate origins of vital forces than with the quality of the acts which stem from them. It sometimes appears that there are some fairly complex behaviours which can and do occur in organisms irrespective of environmental contingencies. One guesses that *some* behaviours or qualities of behaviour depend little on 'learning,' but seem quite innate — even though, as investigated, they are found increasingly to be modifiable or to require certain environmental conditions. In humans, we wonder which of them characterize the species. Modern linguistics leans heavily on the idea that syntax has a neurological substrate. Anthropologically, the wide appeal of Levi Strauss' hypothesis resides in the assumption that, across cultures and races, humans show patterns of behaviour and thought that betray common 'structural' properties. In order to understand anything at all about the biological nature of man's acts, it is these patterns we must be able to distinguish.

An adaptive interactional model will accommodate a huge variety of behavioural events. It frees us from primitive reductionist explanations without, on the other hand, resort to entelechy, teleology, or soul. Psychiatrists know now that even to 'understand' many items of behaviour — there are so many of them, relating in so many subtle and complex ways — does not amount to an understanding of 'behaviour' in any general sense. It is nonetheless possible to apprehend patterns if the organization of behavioural elements is perceived — if we attend to the macro-events as well as the micro-events. In full scale, this includes the concept of a species which exists through evolutionary time. As Hinde has put it: we must ask about a unit of behaviour, what causes it to be there, what is its function, and what is its evolutionary history? Thus, ethology inquires of its subject what the physical sciences cannot, and psychology dare not — that is, what is its purpose? In this way, the addition of a phylogenetic perspective may permit the reformulation of many of psychiatry's major questions.

EARLY DEVELOPMENT

ROBERT A. HINDE

1   Mother/Infant Relations in Rhesus Monkeys*

All those attending this conference, psychiatrists and others, are probably here because of a belief that the proper understanding of human personality development is more important than any of the other problems that face us today, and indeed is basic to most of them. It is a measure of your motivation, or perhaps of your desperation, that you are prepared to attend a meeting in which some of the speakers are not psychiatrists and have never treated human patients. While it is clear that much can be learned from animals about the working of man's physical body, you may feel that his behaviour is a different matter. For example, man's command of language and his superior intellectual development indicate that his behavioural ontogeny is different in kind from that of lower species. It could be argued that the social situation in which man develops is qualitatively different from the social environment in which the infant monkey, for instance, develops. However, there are also similarities. To say that the study of sub-human forms is not useful everywhere is different from saying that it is useful nowhere. This discussion will suggest that studies of lower species can indeed help in understanding the human case — in three ways.

First: Work with animals can be used for the development of techniques for recording behaviour or for simple experiments which are suitable for the human case. There is a growing realization that data on what people actually do, as well as what they say that they do and say that they think, may be important for both clinician and theoretician. Techniques worked out by students of animal behaviour are now being used to this end.

Second: Animals can be used for the study of strictly delimited problems. There are some cases where ethical considerations forbid the relevant experimental techniques with human subjects, and animals must be used — one of

* This work was carried out primarily in collaboration with the late Dr Yvette Spencer-Booth and many of the results were obtained by her. She should be thought of as a joint author of this paper

which is discussed below. In every case the relevance of the animal findings to the human case, must, of course, be tested directly or indirectly at every possible stage.

Third: Studies of animals can lead to new perspectives for the study of behaviour and to the development of principles of behaviour which can then be applied to the human case. Here we are on dangerous ground. The temptation to make slick and easy comparison between animal and man is strong, and some disastrously naive examples are to be found in recent books by Ardrey (1967), Morris (1967), and Lorenz (1966). It is not necessary, however, to fall into that sort of error. To cite but one example, in his recent book on 'Attachment' (1969), Dr John Bowlby has taken up some principles emerging from studies of animals and woven them into a theory of human personal relations which may well have far-reaching repercussions.

There is a specific and well-known problem which shows the relevance of animal studies to man. The research bearing on this which is discussed here was stimulated by Dr John Bowlby's work. Strong evidence has suggested that if a human child is separated for a while from its parents there may be far-reaching effects on its personality. The operative words are 'may be.' Some hold that the effects are never so serious as others make out and, in any case, there are marked individual differences in severity. Furthermore, little is known either about the parameters determining the severity of the effects or about the conditions under which they can be ameliorated. One of the many obstacles to research in this field is that the evidence is so often retrospective, and many potentially important variables are inevitably uncontrolled in human subjects. Since human experimentation is clearly impossible, the question arises: can monkeys be used instead?

It would be absurd to discuss experimental work on the social development of monkeys without reference to the pioneering studies of Dr Harry Harlow (1965) and his colleagues at the University of Wisconsin. His early studies, published about the time this work began, demonstrated the possibility of producing hard quantitative data on something as nebulous as the mother/infant relationships. The work at Wisconsin has had two main themes. First, the question of what makes a good mother for a rhesus monkey infant, showing the importance of contact comfort with surrogate mothers. Second, those factors in the early social environment which are necessary for the development of a 'normal' animal. This latter has involved rearing animals with varying degrees of access to social companions, and has permitted the analysis of social development in terms of five affectional systems: the infant-mother, mother-infant, paternal, peer, and heterosexual systems.

In certain respects the techniques which we have been using have been somewhat different from the earlier ones used at Wisconsin. In his early work

Dr Harlow achieved experimental control by keeping his infants in wire cages which were bare except for the surrogate mother, and attempted to assess the importance of various social factors by adding them one at a time. Feeling something was sacrificed with the resulting impoverishment and artificiality of the environment, it seemed to us desirable to forgo a certain amount of experimental control in order to provide the infants with a social environment that was in some respects similar to that to which their species had evolved. Groups of monkeys were set up, each consisting of a male, two to four females, and subsequently their young. Each group occupied an outside cage eighteen feet long and ten feet high, communicating with an inside room roughly six feet cube. This situation is quite different from that of a natural troop, and is a compromise. We intended *moderate* experimental control, *moderate* precision of recording and, at the same time, a *moderately* complex social environment. There is no suggestion that this method is superior to Harlow's — both approaches appear to be necessary.

PROXIMITY: MAINTENANCE AND CHANGE

All data were collected on check sheets with half-minute time intervals (Figure 1). In each half-minute we recorded such data as whether or not the infant was asleep; whether or not it was on the nipple; or whether it was on the mother but off the nipple; if it was off the mother, whether it was within sixty cm of her or more than sixty cm from her; whether the mother was grooming the baby or the baby was grooming the mother; if the distance between baby and mother changed from more than sixty cm to less or vice versa, we recorded whether it was the mother leaving the baby or the baby leaving the mother, or whether it was the mother approaching the baby or the baby approaching the mother.

The principle measures extracted from the check sheets are as follows. *Total time off the mother* — the number of half-minutes which the infant was off the mother, expressed as a percentage of the number of half-minutes for which it was watched.

Acceptance-rejection — every time the infant attempted to gain the nipple we recorded whether it was accepted or rejected by the mother. We also recorded the occasions on which the infant went on to the nipple on the mother's initiative. This gives us three measures: *Absolute frequency of rejections (R),* the number of times the infant attempted to gain the nipple and was rejected. *Relative frequency of rejections $R/(A+M+R)$,* the ratio of rejections to the total number of times in which it either got on to the nipple, or tried to do so and was rejected. The number of times it got on to the nipple was made up of the number of times it attempted to get on and was accepted *(A)*, and the

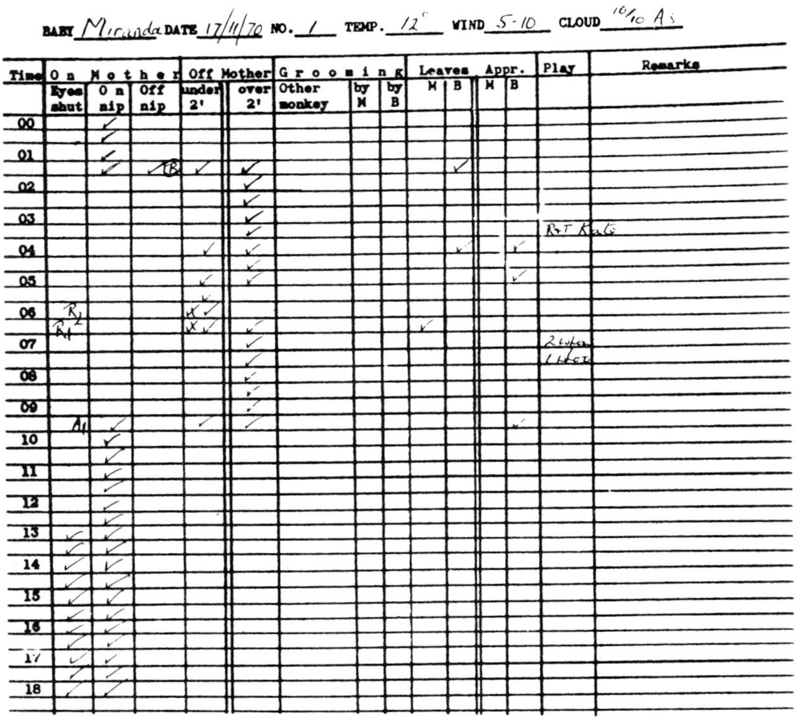

BABY *Miranda* DATE 17/11/70 NO. 1   TEMP. 12°   WIND 5-10   CLOUD 10/10 As

Time	On Mother			Off Mother			Grooming		Leaves		Appr.		Play	Remarks
	Eyes shut	On nip	Off nip	under 2'	over 2'	Other monkey	by M	by B	M	B	M	B		
00		✓												
01		✓												
02		✓	B	✓	✓				✓					
03					✓									
04				✓	✓								R.T KuG	
05					✓						✓			
06	R1			✓	✓									
07	R4			✓	✓	✓			✓				2 6/8 a / H cu	
08					✓									
09					✓									
10	A1	✓		✓										
11		✓												
12		✓												
13	✓	✓												
14	✓	✓												
15	✓	✓												
16	✓	✓												
17	✓	✓												
18	✓	✓												

FIGURE 1   One of the check sheets used in studies of monkey mother/infant interaction

number of times it went on on the mother's initiative *(M). Mother's initiative in nipple contacts M/(A+M)*, the ratio of the number of times that it went on on the mother's initiative to the total number of times that it got on.

Number of half-minutes in which the infant was more than sixty cm from the mother, expressed as a percentage of the total number of half-minutes in which the infant was off the mother. Sixty cm (about two feet) was a distance chosen after some trial and error, and is roughly as far as a mother rhesus can reach in a hurry.

Infant's role in maintaining proximity to the mother. As mentioned above, on every occasion that the distance between mother and infant changed from more than to less than sixty cm, or vice versa, it was recorded whether it was the mother or infant approaching, or the mother or infant leaving. From that was calculated the proportion of approaches and the proportion of leavings that were due to the infant. The difference between these two – the

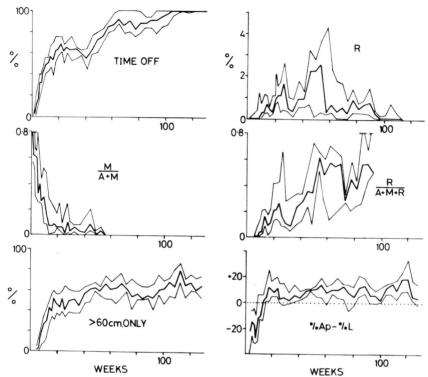

FIGURE 2   Age changes in mother/infant interaction. Medians and interquartile ranges for *N* = 16 (weeks 1-24) or 8 (weeks 24-130)
Top left: no. of ½-min in which off mother as percentage of no. of occasions observed
Top right: no. of times infant attempted to gain nipple and was rejected per 100 x ½ min (*R*)
Centre left: maternal initiative in nipple contacts. *M* (no. of times infants were picked up by mothers)/[*A* (no. of times infants were accepted by mothers) + *M*]
Centre right: relative frequency of rejections: $R/A + M + R$
Bottom left: no. of ½-min which infants spent wholly more than 60 cm from their mothers as percentage of no. in which they were off her
Bottom right: infant initiative in maintaining proximity. Percentage of approaches (*Ap*) due to infant, minus percentage of leavings (*L*) due to infant

percentage of approaches minus the percentage of leavings — gives a measure of the infant's role in maintaining proximity to its mother. If this is positive, it means that the infant is responsible for a higher proportion of approaches than it is of leavings, and thus that the infant is primarily responsible for maintaining proximity.

Figure 2 shows some examples of the use of these measures in recording mother/infant interaction over the first two-and-one-half years of life. Each graph is based on about ten infants that were watched for six hours a week, six hours a fortnight, or six hours a month, according to the age of the infant. All the watches were made in the morning hours. The thick line in each case is the median, and the thin lines on either side show the interquartile range. The time off the mother increases to a plateau towards the end of the first year, and then in the second year increases up to one hundred per cent. The next three measures are concerned with the role of mother and infant in determining how much time the infant spends off its mother. The absolute frequency of rejections rises to a peak about the end of the first year and then falls off again. That the falling-off is due to decreasing demand by the infant is shown by the relative frequency of rejections, which goes on increasing and stays high up to the point at which rejections are so rare that it can no longer be measured reliably. The mother's role in initiating nipple contact falls off fairly rapidly during the first few months of life.

The proportion of its time off the mother that the infant spends more than sixty cm from her increases up to about sixty or seventy per cent at the end of the first year and then only slowly thereafter. The measure of the infant's role in maintaining proximity to its mother is negative during the first twenty weeks, indicating that the infant is responsible for a higher proportion of leavings than it is of approaches. Thus it is the mother who is primarily responsible for maintaining proximity to the infant. After the infant is about twenty weeks old this measure becomes positive and remains so thereafter, indicating that from that age it is the infant who is primarily responsible for keeping near its mother.

These measures are concerned with the nature of the mother/infant relationship, and with the roles of mother and infant in determining the nature of that relationship, at each age. A second problem concerns the roles of *changes* in the behaviour of mother and infant in determining the age changes in their relationship. In order to assess this we must look, not at the measures themselves, but at the relationships between the measures. A convenient starting point is to consider how far the observed changes in the mother/infant relationship can be understood as the effects of one or more of four possible simple types of change in the participants – namely an increase or a decrease in the tendencies of either mother or infant to respond positively (i.e., other than by avoidance or aggression) to the other.

These are shown in Table I. For each of these possibilities one can predict what will happen to each of the measures of the mother/infant relationship. If the infant tends to leave the mother more, then time off the mother will increase; the absolute and relative frequency of rejections will decrease; the relative role of the mother in initiating nipple contacts will increase; the time

TABLE I Predicted direction of changes in various measures of mother-infant inter-action produced by four simple types of change in the behaviour of one of them

	Time off mother	Relative frequency of rejections $R/(A+M+R)$	Time at a distance from mother >60 cms	Infant's role in maintaining proximity $\% Ap - \% L$
Infant leaves mother more	+	−	+	−
Infant seeks proximity more	−	+	−	+
Mother seeks proximity more	−	−	−	−
Mother leaves infant more	+	+	+	+

spent at a distance from the mother will increase; the percentage of approaches by the infant will increase, and of arithmetical necessity, the measure of the infant's role in maintaining proximity will decrease. In this way, predictions for each of the four possibilities shown on the left of Table I can be made. If the changes in mother/infant interaction could, in fact, be understood simply in terms of those simple changes shown on the left hand side of Table I, then certain measures of the mother/infant interaction would always be correlated with each other. For instance, time off the mother always changes in the same direction as the proportion of that time spent at a distance from the mother. Similarly, the frequency of rejections would always be correlated with the infant's role in maintaining proximity. There-fore, the extent to which these pairs of measures are in fact correlated with each other is a measure of the extent to which changes in the mother/infant relationship can be understood in terms of the four simple changes.

Table I also makes it possible to separate the relative roles of changes in the mother's behaviour and changes in the infant's behaviour in determining changes in the nature of their relationship. For instance, if the time off the mother increases this could be due to a change in the infant's behaviour, or to a change in the mother's behaviour. If it is immediately due to a change in the infant's behaviour, it will be negatively correlated with the frequency of rejections. If it is due to a change in the mother's behaviour, it will be positively correlated with the frequency of rejections. Similarly, if the time spent at a distance from the mother increases, it will be immediately due to a change in the infant's behaviour if it is negatively correlated with the measure of the infant's role in maintaining proximity, and to a change in the mother's behaviour if positively correlated.

Table II illustrates this in practice. Since visual examination indicated that the mother/infant relationship changed with age, correlation coefficients were calculated separately for weeks one to six, weeks seven to twenty, and weeks twenty-one and thereafter. Rejections were so infrequent in the early weeks

TABLE II Spearman rank order correlation coefficients between median values of measures for all individuals in each age span. From upper left to lower right figures refer to weeks 1-6 ($N = 6$), weeks 7-20 ($N = 7$), and weeks 21 on. Rejections were rare in the early period

	$R/(A+M+R)$	>60 cm	$\% Ap - \% L$
Time off	$\cdots$ +0.54 +0.69†	+0.98† +0.96† +74†	+0.96† +0.94† +0.38*
$R/A+M+R$		$\cdots$ +0.50 +0.57†	$\cdots$ +0.36 +0.63*
60 cm			+0.79 +0.93† +0.57†

* Statistically significant at 0.05 level
† Statistically significant at 0.01 level

that correlations involving them could not be calculated. The time the infant spent off its mother and the relative frequency of rejections were positively correlated, as were the time the infant spent at a distance from its mother and the infant's role in maintaining proximity. From Table I, such positive correlations indicate that the mother is immediately responsible for the increase, with age, in the time that the infant spends off and at a distance from its mother.

This finding is surprising because, to the naive observer, the increasing independence of the infant is associated with (and seems to be an immediate consequence of) its increasing strength and locomotor ability. This analysis indicates that changes in the mother's behaviour play a major role in the increasing independence of the infant. This is the case even during those first twenty weeks when it is the mother who is primarily responsible for maintaining proximity to the infant. This indicates that the questions 'Who is responsible for maintaining proximity?' and 'Changes in whose behaviour are responsible for age-changes in proximity?' are different questions. During the first twenty weeks it is the mother who is primarily responsible for maintaining proximity, but it is also changes in the mother's behaviour which are immediately responsible for the increasing independence of the infant. Of course, change in the mother's behaviour to the infant may be initiated by changes in the infant's behaviour, such as its increasing demand for milk or its increasing play behaviour — and these are consequences of its development, which in turn depends on the mother. The changes in the relationship with age must, of course, involve complex interactions between mother and infant,

TABLE IIIA Days of data collection for 6-day separation experiments. On each of these days the infant was watched from 1000 hr until it had been off its mother for a total of 2 hr, or until 1430 hr, whichever was the earlier. Data on mother/infant inter-action and infant activity off the mother was collected. For some aspects of the subsequent analysis, post-separation data were lumped as shown by the dashed lines. Before and after this experimental period routine data on mother/infant interaction were collected for 6 hr a week, fortnight, or month, according to the age of the infant

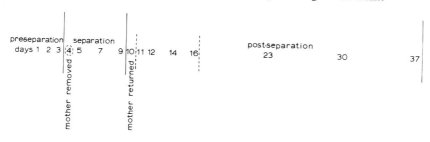

FIGURE IIIB Scheme of separation experiments

	N	21weeks	25–26weeks	30–32weeks
Single Separation	5			6days
Two Separations(1)	5+1	6days		6days
Two Separations(2)	5		6days	6days
Long Separation	6			13days

SEPARATION GROUPS

but this analysis shows that the mother's role in not only permitting, but also promoting, the infant's independence must not be underestimated.

THE EFFECTS OF SEPARATION

The effects of a period of separation from the mother have now been studied by a number of investigators. The data considered here will be confined to those taken from our own work. In our initial experiments we investigated the effects of removing the mother from the home pen for six days when the infant was thirty to thirty-two weeks old. The exact equivalent of this in

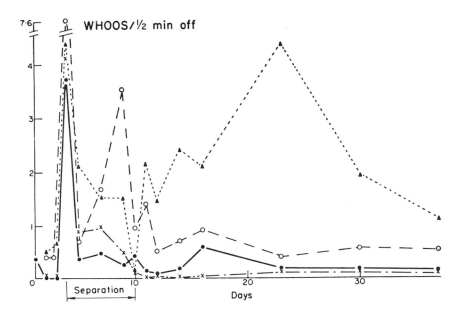

FIGURE 3   The mean number of whoo-calls per ½ min spent off mother during the experimental period. Each line represents a different individual

human age is impossible to estimate, but we were guided by wanting to remove the mothers when the infants were as young as possible, while still being certain that they could support themselves without their mothers. Later we found we could work with somewhat younger infants. Since the mothers were removed it was essentially a 'mother goes to hospital' rather than an 'infant goes to hospital' situation. Table IIIA shows the design of the experiments. The figures represent the days, from the start of our observations, on which data were collected. Day four is the day on which the mothers were removed and day ten that on which they were returned. Observations were continued for a month after the return of the mothers. Figures show individual data for the first four infants. Figure 3 shows the distress calling of the infants – the analogue of human crying. This increased enormously when the mothers were removed, and slowly decreased thereafter; but in each of these four infants the amount of 'whoo' calling was still higher a month after the mother was returned than it had been before she had been removed. Soon after the mothers' removal the infants became very depressed. They shuffled around with their heads shrunk on their shoulders and just looked miserable.

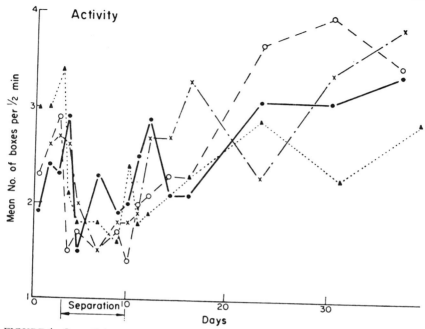

FIGURE 4 Over-all locomotor activity of infants when off mother during the experimental period. The run was divided into 16 'boxes,' and the ordinate gives the mean number entered per ½-minute

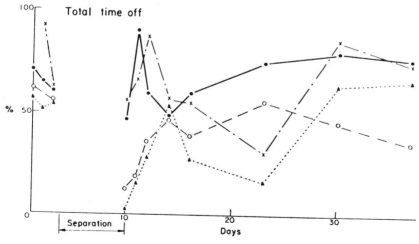

FIGURE 5 The percentage of ½ minutes in which the infants were recorded off their mothers during the experimental period

This is exemplified by a measure of locomotor ability: the cage was divided into sixteen sections and the mean number which the infants entered per half-minute period was calculated. Figure 4 shows that while the mothers were away the locomotor ability dropped markedly, and then on their return recovered. Figure 5 shows the time spent off the mothers, and it can be seen that after the mother was returned, two of the infants became very clinging indeed and spent very little time off their mothers. This gradually recovered with time, though in all four of these infants the recovery was not simple — it involved a period of temporary recovery, then regression, and then a more permanent recovery. Each infant showed this sort of biphasic recovery. The type of analysis indicated in Table I showed that this biphasic recovery was a consequence of a complex interaction between mother and infant in the immediately post-separation period. This may be very important in determining the ultimate nature of the effects of the separation.

The conspicuous feature of the data for these four infants was the large individual variability. In an attempt to pinpoint the variables which influenced the effect of the separation experience, we carried out separation experiments as shown in Table IIIB. The programme included three groups who were given a six-day separation experience at either twenty-one weeks, twenty-five weeks, or thirty weeks. Within this age-range the age of separation made very little difference, and the changes in behaviour were similar to those shown in Figures 4-6. In addition to the measures already mentioned, the frequency of tantrums, low while the mother was away, became high on the day that she returned; the frequency with which the infant was recorded sitting doing nothing (which is, in some but not all respects, the inverse of activity) increased while the mother was away and then subsequently returned to normal; and both manipulative and rough-and-tumble play decreased very markedly in the mother's absence. The measure of the infant's role in maintaining proximity increased when the mother was returned, indicating that the infant was making great demands on the mother.

In these experiments the length of the separation period was six days, but another group was given a thirteen-day separation period at thirty to thirty-two weeks. As shown in Table IIIB the design permitted comparison of the effects of (i) a single separation of six days, (ii) the second of two six-day separation periods, and (iii) a single separation of thirteen days, at thirty to thirty-two weeks. After a thirteen-day separation the measures of mother/infant interaction differed little from those after one or two six-day separation periods, but there were consistent differences in the measures of the infant's behaviour off the mother. Those infants who were separated from their mothers for the longer period showed least activity and most whoo-

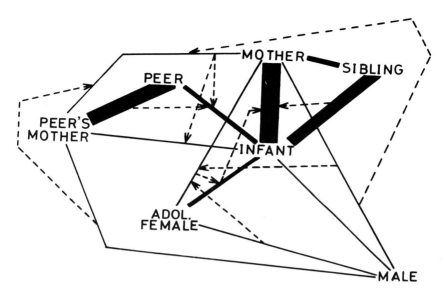

FIGURE 6 Schematic representation of the social nexus in which the infant is im-
bedded. Continuous lines represent inter-individual relationships, their thickness giving a
subjective impression of their importance. Discontinuous lines represent effects of one
relationship on another

calling during the month after the mother's return. This finding shows that
the effects of a separation experience have parametric properties.

The same marked individual variation which we found in the initial experiments at thirty to thirty-two weeks was present in all groups. Analysis of the
data showed that three of the variables which might have been expected to
influence the effects of the separation experience had, in fact, only a minor
effect. These were: the age of the infant (within this range); the dominance
status of the mother within the group in which she was living; and the
amount of attention which the infant got from other group companions
during the mother's absence. There was, however, a slight tendency for male
infants to be affected more than female.

NATURE OF THE RELATIONSHIP

Another possible factor of importance in determining the severity of the
effects is the nature of the mother/infant relationship. To pursue this
question it was necessary to assess how much the individual infants were

disturbed by the separation experience in terms of measures which had nothing to do with the mother/infant relationship itself. To this end we used the measures of locomotor activity, of the frequency with which the infants were recorded sitting doing nothing, and of the rate of whoo-calling, all measures which were markedly affected by the separation experience. These measures were positively but not always significantly correlated with each other, some infants being affected markedly in showing, for instance, a high rate of distress calling, and other infants, for instance, in showing low locomotor activity. We therefore combined these three measures by calculating a 'distress index' which involved summing the ranks of the infants on all three. This 'distress index' was, in fact, correlated highly during the post-separation period with the frequency with which the infants showed tantrums.

These distress indices showed high inter-correlations between the different parts of the experiment. That those infants most distressed after the mother's return were also those most distressed before her removal indicates that the effect of the separation experience was to enhance pre-existing but small individual differences between the infants.

We used this distress index to see whether an infant's response to separation was related to the nature of the mother/infant relationship, looking first for correlations between the distress index and contemporaneous measures of the mother/infant relationship. Table IV shows rank order correlation coefficients between the distress index before separation, on the day that the mother was returned, and during two subsequent post-separation periods, with the contemporaneous measures of the mother/infant relationship. There was very little correlation before separation. This was perhaps related to the fact that all infants were actually showing very little distress anyway, so that the distress index was much more influenced by random effects of sampling. Nor was there any correlation on the day the mother went back, when complex interactions between mother and infant occur. But in the two subsequent periods the distress index was weakly negatively correlated with time off the mother, indicating that those infants who spent least time off the mother were most distressed. Of greater interest were the strong correlations between the distress index and both the amount the infant was rejected by the mother and the role it had to play in staying near the mother. Speaking colloquially, it seemed as though the distress index was related not so much to how much time the mother and infant spent together, but rather to how much 'tension' there was in their relationship.

These measures of the mother/infant relationship were correlated between the pre-separation and post-separation periods. We therefore examined the extent to which the distress index *after* separation was related to the

TABLE IV Spearman rank order correlation coefficients between distress index in post-separation watches and contemporaneous measures of mother/infant interaction

DISTRESS INDEX ON

CONTEMP.	Pre-sep	Day 10	Day 11-16	Day 23-37
Time off	·01	−·09	−·39	−·37
R/A+M+R	−·08	·18	·51[+]	·59[+]
>2ft	−·14	·08	−·58[+]	·11
%Ap.−%L	·14	·22	·51[+]	·45[+]

Spearman rank order correlation coefficients

TABLE V Spearman rank order correlation coefficients between distress index in post-separation watches and pre-separation measures of mother/infant interaction

DISTRESS INDEX ON

PRE-SEP.	DAY 10	DAY 11-16	DAY 23-37
Time off	·02	−·07	−·13
R/A+M+R	·41	·59[+]	·43[+]
>2ft	−·26	−·28	−·18
%Ap.−%L	·30	·64[++]	·41

Spearman rank order correlation coefficients

measures of the mother/infant relationship *before* separation. The correlation coefficients are shown in Table v, and present a similar picture: the distress index after separation, at any rate after day ten, was related to the frequency of rejections and to the role of the infant in maintaining proximity before separation.

The next question was: is the distress after separation more closely related to the mother/infant relationship before separation, or to the contemporaneous mother/infant relationship? For this, instead of using Spearman rank order correlation coefficients, it was necessary to use Kendall tau partial correlation coefficients. These showed that the distress index immediately after separation was strongly related to the pre-separation mother/infant relationship, but that as time elapsed the amount of distress shown became less related to what had happened before separation and more related to the contemporaneous nature of the mother/infant relationship.

Although these data show that the effect of the period of maternal separation is at least related to the nature of the preceding mother/infant relationship, we cannot, strictly speaking, say that the nature of the mother/infant relationship determines the response to separation: our correlations could mean merely that those infants with a particular sort of mother/infant relationship were those most likely to be affected by a separation experience. However, a causal relationship at least seems likely.

PERSISTENCE OF EFFECTS

Finally, we have tried to assess the durability of the effects of a separation experience. We have given the infants a series of rather simple-minded tests at various intervals after the separation experience. These tests include examining the characteristics of the mother/infant relationship; recording the locomotor and play activity of the infants; measuring their readiness to approach strange objects or to take vitamin pills from the experimenter; looking at their responses to mildly frustrating situations like a date hanging just out of reach.

Since the results involve a variety of tests they are difficult to summarize adequately. The main series was carried out when the infants were a year old, i.e., five to six months after the separation experience. When tested in their home cage at this age, or when they were moved to a strange cage, there were only minor differences in the mother/infant relationship between control animals which had had no separation experience and those which had had one or two six-day separation experiences. Furthermore, when tested in their home cage for their readiness to approach a mirror with grass in front of it, or to approach a banana, there were no significant differences between the controls and the animals which had had one or two separation experiences. There were, however, significant differences in their readiness to approach the experimenter, who had been responsible for removing their mothers six months previously, to get vitamins. There were also differences in their activity, those which had had a separation experience tending to sit more and to show less locomotor activity. They also showed less social play and more manipulative play than the animals which had had no separation experience. When tested in a *strange* cage for their approaches to strange objects, the previously separated animals differed significantly from the controls in a large number of ways, being more upset or less ready to approach.

Even five to six months afterwards there were thus still marked differences between those animals which had had no separation experience and those which had. Further tests carried out when the infants were two-and-a-half years old, i.e., two years after the separation experience, again yielded a number of significant differences between the controls and the experimentals when they were tested in a strange situation, though these were less dramatic than in the tests at twelve months.

USE OF THE DATA

I began by discussing the relevance to man of studies of sub-human species. The final judgment on this issue must be in the hands not of students of animal behaviour, but of the human psychologists and psychiatrists. All that students of animal behaviour can do is to offer them the data, and they must see what use they can make of them. Nonetheless, I do submit that we have here a particular effect in man which can be reproduced in monkeys – and, allowing for the species differences, the symptoms shown after a separation experience are very similar in monkey and in man. The only major difference seems to be that the phase of detachment, or rejection of the mother by the infant after the separation experience, is not present in monkeys – at any rate, not to the same extent as in man. If the symptoms are similar in man and in prelinguistic monkey, this in itself places limits on the complexity of the explanatory hypotheses that are necessary in the human case. The data presented here also go a little way towards making possible a prognosis about which infant monkeys will, or will not, be severely affected by such an experience. Similar factors may also be important in man. I am aware, of course, that the psychiatrists may say: 'Of course we knew that the nature of the mother/infant relationship was the important predetermining factor,' but I hope that quantitative data will help to allay the subconscious doubts to which I believe even psychiatrists are susceptible, and that they will also help to pinpoint precisely which aspects of the mother/infant relationship are important. And finally, I believe we have demonstrated that the effects of the separation experience may be rather long lasting — and if they are long lasting in monkeys, it seems likely that they will also be in man.

I. CHARLES KAUFMAN

2 Mother/Infant Relations in Monkeys and Humans: A Reply to Professor Hinde*

Having had the privilege of studying with Professor Hinde for a year in the late 1950s I was prepared for his impressive presentation: first, of the rationale for animal behaviour studies and their relevance to the human; second, of his own sound methodological, reasoned progression of experimental studies; and third, of his sophisticated, yet simple and therefore elegant, statistical analysis of the data.

In this work, Professor Hinde has addressed himself to very important topics. For humans, and all higher organisms, life begins with a long period during which independent functioning is not possible, and normal development depends upon continuous parental care. The nature of that care and its effect on the developing infant are obviously of fundamental importance. In primates the work of elucidating the variable involved using three paradigms: naturalistic studies in the field; experimental studies in the laboratory; and semi-naturalistic studies of created, contained, or otherwise controlled social groups. Each has its unique advantages, and each has obvious disadvantages. All are required for the total study of the questions involved.

Professor Hinde has used the semi-natural approach to great advantage in studying, first, the mother/infant interaction and its role in infant development in a social setting, and then the effect of mother-loss. He has pointed out that observers disagree about the seriousness of parent-loss in the human, but we realize that most have looked at very different examples of it — the monstrous deprivation of a Kaspar-Hauser, or mother going to hospital, or child going to hospital, or to school, or left with a sitter for an afternoon, and so on. That is, the effects of mother-loss, both short-term and long-term, depend on a variety of factors: the age, or developmental level; a related factor, the availability and adequacy of coping mechanisms; the length of the loss; the personal, experiential meaning of the loss; the availability and

* The research for this paper was supported by grants MH-04670 and -18144 from the National Institute of Mental Health, US Public Health Service, Bethesda, Md.

adequacy of substitute mothering; the presence of additional stresses; individual variation based on constitutional and experiential determinants; and others. Furthermore, what observers see depends on *when* they look – and also on the *stages* of reaction to separation. In any case, there is no doubt that dramatic and deleterious consequences do frequently follow mother-loss, and Professor Hinde's work both demonstrates some of these and helps explain them, in monkeys at least.

Let us consider some details of his paper. Rhesus macaques were put together in relatively spacious enclosures, where they bred, and were systematically observed, noting the frequency of each behaviour. Other investigators have used similar techniques and compiled comparable kinds of data: for example, on the amount of time the infant is on the mother, or off, or away; on the approaches or departures by mother when the infant approaches; and so on. The data from a number of laboratories on several species of macaque agree in essence that early in life mother and infant are very close, that there is then a stage in which efforts by the infant to disengage are frequently thwarted by the mother, but that then there is a progressive physical separation of the pair, with the infant spending more and more time away from mother, engaged in play behaviour, increasingly with peers. An important question has been – how come? Is this increasing separation an autonomous development of independence in the infant? Or is the mother, so to speak, chasing him away? Using the measures mentioned above, various observers have found support for both views.

Professor Hinde has ingeniously carried his analysis one step further by examining the relations *between* measures, using a conceptual model of *expected* relations between measures in four polar conditions of mother/ infant relations – mother behaves positively, mother does not behave positively, infant behaves positively, infant does not behave positively. It could be argued that this model oversimplifies in that, by examining the role of each partner, the *interaction between them* may be lost sight of, a possibility that Professor Hinde recognizes. Furthermore, it does not take into account more ultimate causes of behaviour. Professor Hinde and others have shown that dyadic relations are strongly influenced by the presence or absence of other animals, and by other aspects of the environment.

Be that as it may, let us look at his interesting findings. As the first year of life unfolds and the infant shows increasing non-filial activity, he finds two strong positive correlations between behavioural measures; one is between time off mother and frequency of maternal rejections; and the second is between time at a distance from mother and the infant's efforts in maintaining proximity. His explanation is that, however caused, the increased estrangement of the dyad is due to the mother not behaving positively, i.e., to her rejecting behaviour. When we examine his studies of mother-loss again we shall see the potent effect of maternal rejection.

In his separation studies he removed the mothers for varying periods of time, leaving the infants, of varying ages, in their usual surroundings. A number of factors were found *not* to influence the infant's reaction – the infant's age, the infant's sex, the mother's dominance status, and the infant's interaction with other animals. One wonders about a factor which is not mentioned – the size of the social group – since the groups were of variable size, a factor that may influence mother/infant interaction. He *did* find that the extent of separation played a role, since the effects were greater with repeated and longer separations.

The infants showed a marked reaction to mother-loss, with distress and depression. They vocalized a great deal, showed a marked drop in activity, and sat around a lot doing nothing. When the mother returned there was a resumption of closeness. However, there was considerable individual variation in the reaction during separation and after reunion. To get at this variability he devised a distress index as an over-all measure of the infant's reaction.

In correlating the distress index with aspects of the mother/infant relationship, he found nothing significant on the day of reunion, but thereafter there were significant findings. The most distressed infants were those who, both before and after separation, were the most rejected despite greater efforts to approach mother. Professor Hinde concludes that the degree of distress in response to mother-loss is based on 'tension' in the relationship, both before the separation and after reunion. He thus provides corroboration in the monkey for our clinical impression in humans that the nature of the mother/infant relationship affects the way in which an infant reacts to loss of mother.

In his follow-up studies he provides evidence that an experience of separation from mother has long-lasting disturbing effects, particularly anxiety when confronted by unfamiliarity. These are all important findings with obvious relevance to the human situation. First, with respect to normal development Professor Hinde has stressed the important role of maternal rejection in the increasing separation of the mother/infant dyad, but his data also show a strong correlation between maternal rejection and efforts by the infant to reach mother, efforts which we must assume to be a measure of the infant's dependence or attachment. The relation between rejection and attraction need not surprise us if we consider the techniques of the seductress. To be less clinical, we may recall Hess' (1959) demonstration that the harder a baby bird has to follow a mother figure the more strongly imprinted it becomes. Also, Harlow and Rosenblum (1963) showed that the more a surrogate mother rejected a monkey infant by blasting him with air, the tighter the

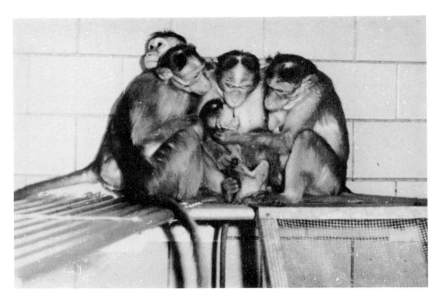

FIGURE 1   A group of bonnet females in a huddle, including a mother and her young
infant, who is the centre of interest. (From I.C. Kaufman and L.A. Rosenblum, Effects
of separation from mother on the emotional behavior of infant monkeys. *Ann. NY Acad.
Sci.* 159 (1969), 681-95)

infant clung. Within limits, then, rejection generally leads to an increase in
dependency behaviour. This is one reason for questioning the overriding role
of maternal rejection in effecting the infant's *independence.* There are, however, other reasons. J.H. Kaufman (1966), in a field study of rhesus monkeys
concluded re independence that 'Rejection of the infant seemed insignificant
compared to the infant's interest in other monkeys, especially other infants.'
In chimpanzees, Goodall (1965) found little rejection by the mother, but a
rather consistent initiative by the infant with respect to exploration and
interactions with peers and older juveniles. In humans, Mahler (1968) has
stressed the child's drive toward independence in her studies of separation-
individuation. Studies in my laboratory also tend to favour the thesis that the
growing primate has a very considerable exploratory and do-it-yourself tendency which is largely responsible for his growing independence (Kaufman
and Rosenblum, 1969).

For nine years we have been studying numerous groups of two species of
macaque, pigtails and bonnets. This work has been done largely in collaboration with L.A. Rosenblum and A.J. Stynes. Although taxonomically close
(Kaufman and Rosenblum, 1966), and sharing many behaviours and social
characteristics, we found some striking differences between these two species.

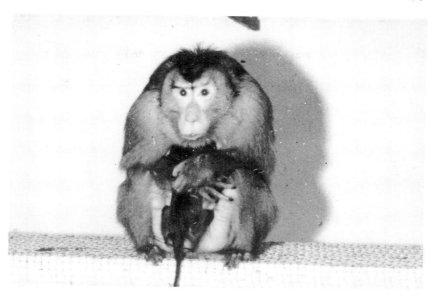

FIGURE 2 A pigtail mother, alone on a shelf with her young infant, showing threat behaviour. (From I.C. Kaufman and L.A. Rosenblum, Effects of separation from mother on the emotional behavior of infant monkeys. *Ann. NY Acad. Sci.* 159 (1969), 681-95)

Bonnet adults tend to remain physically close, often in huddles, whereas pigtails do not usually make physical contact with neighbours except to engage in dynamic social interactions such as grooming, mating, or fighting. At night, pigtails tend to sleep lying down, whereas bonnets tend to sleep sitting up, maintaining physical contact with each other. Since this difference has been manifested by every group we have formed, utilizing animals captured at different times, and probably in different places, we must assume that this is a species difference. How this difference arose is not known at this time, but its consequences upon social organization and upon infant rearing are of considerable interest.

The tendency to propinquity among the bonnets continues during pregnancy and after the delivery of the young when bonnet females return to close contact (Figure 1), whereas pigtail females with infants tend to remain apart (Figure 2) from other females. Both provide their infants with the intensive maternal care which characterizes primates, but the bonnet mother does it alongside of her peers whereas the pigtail mother does it in relative isolation. The bonnet mother allows other females to pay considerable attention to her infant and even to interact with it, whereas the pigtail mother tends to guard jealously her infant from the attentions of others. As a result,

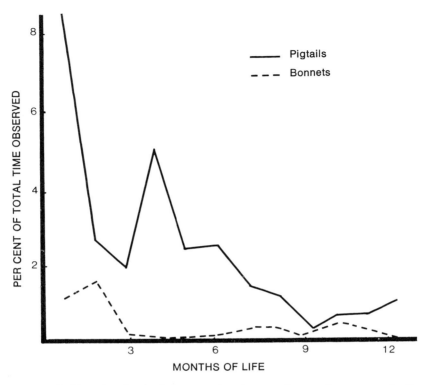

FIGURE 3 Mean duration in the two species of maternal protectiveness over the first year of life. This index represents the combined scores for departure restraint, guard, retrieval, and watch. (From I.C. Kaufman and L.A. Rosenblum, Effects of separation from mother on the emotional behavior of infant monkeys. *Ann. NY Acad. Sci.* 159 (1969), 681-95)

bonnet infants, even in the first month of life, have significantly more social interactions with animals other than their mothers than do pigtail infants.

In the next few months, infants in both species tend to initiate separations from their mothers. In virtually all dyads of both species that we have observed, it is the infant that initiates, from early on, most of the breaks in contact. The initial breaks are quite brief, and the infant, guarded closely by the mother, does not venture far from her. There is then a gradual increase in the amount of time spent away from the mother, but still on the same level of the pen. During the first several months, however, the mother rarely eases to watch intently her separated infant. Indeed, the infant is often *retrieved* in an instant in response to stimuli perceived by the mother but often undetected by the observer. Mothers of both species show other protective

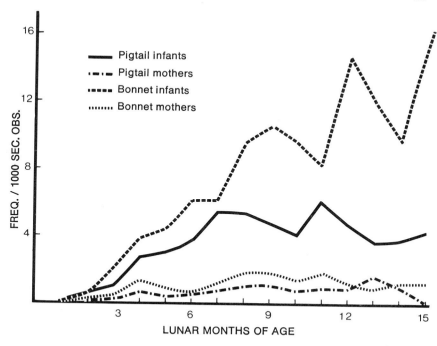

FIGURE 4   The relative frequency of vertical departures by mothers and infants in pigtail and bonnet dyads. (From I.C. Kaufman and L.A. Rosenblum, The waning of the mother-infant bond in two species of macaque. In B. Foss (ed.), *Determinants of Infant Behaviour,* vol. 4. London: Methuen, 1969)

behaviours as well, such as restraining the infant from leaving, or guarding him as he moves about. Pigtail mothers show considerably more protective behaviour than bonnets (Figure 3).

Beginning in the second month of life, the infants begin to move to other levels of the pen, leaving their mothers behind. The frequency and duration of these *vertical departures* increase dramatically after the first month and reach a high asymptotic level at about the eighth month. It is clear (Figure 4) that it is the infants who are primarily responsible for these separations. Consideration of the frequency and total duration of these maximum separations between mother and infant provides the first evidence of a distinction between bonnet and pigtail infants developing in our laboratory. From about the third month of life onward, bonnet infants consistently spend more time than pigtails at different levels of the pen than their mothers, apparently reflecting a greater relative security of bonnet infants in their physical and

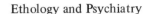

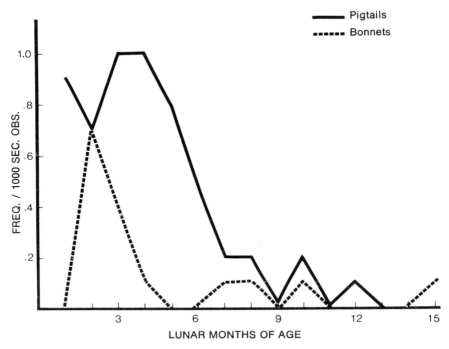

FIGURE 5   The relative frequency of *retrieval* by pigtail and bonnet mothers during the first 15 months of their infant's life. (From I.C. Kaufman and L.A. Rosenblum, The waning of the mother-infant bond in two species of macaque. In B. Foss (ed.), *Determinants of Infant Behaviour,* vol. 4. London: Methuen, 1969)

social environment, and a real difference in their dependence upon mother as they mature. In this regard, it is of interest to note that retrieval, reflecting as it does maternal apprehension over the welfare of the separated infant, appears considerably less often, peaks earlier and wanes more rapidly in bonnet as compared to pigtail mothers (Figure 5). The lesser degree of retrieval by bonnet mothers is undoubtedly related to the greater degree of maximum separation shown by bonnet infants; the mothers allow the infants to go — and they go.

    In both species as maternal solicitude wanes, there is a tendency for the mothers to be less restrictive of their infants, to encourage them to depart, and even to prevent them from returning. This tendency is manifested primarily by weaning and punitive behaviours. In both of these behaviours bonnet mothers show an earlier peak than pigtail mothers (i.e., they stop sooner), and a considerably lower frequency (Figure 6).

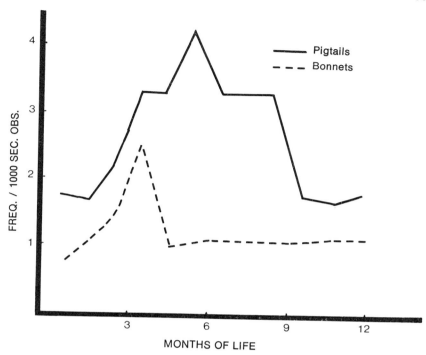

FIGURE 6 Frequency of maternal abdyadic behaviour in the two species over the first year of life. This index represents the combined occurrence of weaning, punitive deterrence, infant removal, and contact-deterrence. (From I.C. Kaufman and L.A. Rosenblum, Effects of separation from mother on the emotional behavior of infant monkeys. *Ann. NY Acad. Sci.* 159 (1969), 681-95)

To recapitulate, the bonnet mother retrieves and protects less, weans less, and punishes less. She appears to allow, but not necessarily to coerce, the developing freedom and independence of her offspring.

In both species, overlapping the changing pattern of mother/infant inter-action, is the continuously increasing interest of the growing infant in his peers and in the environment about him. The infant's growing dexterity and co-ordination is coupled with his increasing freedom of departure from the mother, as her restraining and protective behaviours diminish. Rather rapidly, the initially tentative and hesitant movements away from mother emerge into energetic solitary play activities, which we term *exercise play*. These playful behaviours then become increasingly focused on peers, and *social play* soon becomes the most prominent non-filial activity. Although the total time spent

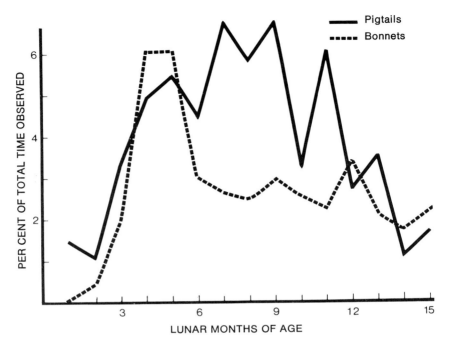

FIGURE 7 Mean duration of *exercise play* in pigtail and bonnet infants during the first 15 months of life. (From I.C. Kaufman and L.A. Rosenblum, The waning of the mother-infant bond in two species of macaque. In B. Foss (ed.), *Determinants of Infant Behaviour*, vol. 4. London: Methuen, 1969)

in play in the two species is the same, the pigtail infants show more *exercise play* (Figure 7), whereas bonnets show more *social play* (Figure 8).

It is apparent that a developmental distinction exists between bonnet and pigtail dyads. The tendency towards closeness between bonnet adults seems to be reflected in a relatively relaxed maternal disposition. Bonnet mothers are less likely to retrieve their separated infants than are pigtail mothers. Similarly, bonnet mothers seem more tolerant of the continued closeness of their growing infants, weaning and punishing them less often. As a consequence, the bonnet infant appears to be more secure: it is less dependent on its mother than the pigtail, in that it leaves her more often and goes further away; it is freer to approach other members of the group, both adults and peers; and it spends more time in social play, whereas the pigtail infant spends more time in exercise play. In the mothers' behaviour and the infants' development, we may see a mechanism of great consequence in the

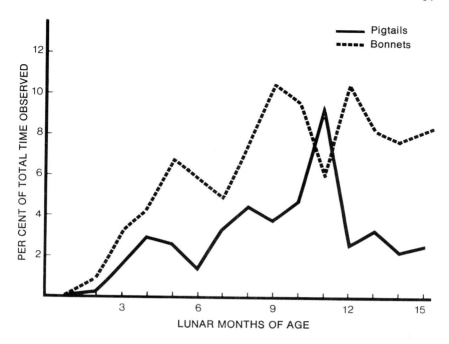

FIGURE 8   Mean duration of *social play* in pigtail and bonnet infants during the first 15 months of life. (From I.C. Kaufman and L.A. Rosenblum, The waning of the mother-infant bond in two species of macaque. In B. Foss (ed.), *Determinants of Infant Behaviour,* vol. 4. London: Methuen, 1969)

perpetuation of the species-characteristic difference in spatial patterning and temperament. Since the difference between these species undoubtedly arose in response to selective pressures, it is reasonable to assume that this difference is genetically encoded. Yet we can see how it becomes realized ontogenetically under the influence of differential mothering patterns of behaviour. This may be another example of nature's redundancy in ensuring selected patterns of behaviour. As Washburn and Hamburg (1965) put it, learning is part of the adaptive pattern of a species, and evolution through selection has built the biological base so that the proper behaviours for that species are the ones that are easily learned.

What do these data contribute to a consideration of the relative contribution of maternal rejection to the ultimate independence of the infant? Comparison of the developmental trends in the two species does not support the idea that maternal rejection is *the* important determinant of the growing independence of the young. Bonnet mothers reject their infants far less often than do pigtail mothers. Yet, judging by the amount of time spent maximally separated from the mother, and in play with peers, both important measures of relative independence, bonnet infants by the end of the first year seem less dependent on their mothers than do pigtails.

It would appear, then, that factors other than maternal rejection per se must be taken into account in considering the waning of the mother/infant bond in macaques. As the processes of physical growth and maturation proceed, and the sensorimotor apparatus elaborates and differentiates, the infant progressively engages his environment. His emerging interest in his social environment is subject to various influences, including the increasing freedom of movement over space and time and in social interaction that is allowed by the mother, a social preference for peers, and the unrestricted availability of peers in a varied environment. The powerful influence of maternal behaviour is seen in the differential rate of development of independence, the bonnet mothers fostering independence not through rejection but through freedom and security.

Let us examine further the role of maternal rejection. Our data, and that of Rosenblum and Harlow, mentioned above, suggest that intermittent rejection by the mother seems to *increase,* rather than decrease, the infant's dependency and his desire for what Harlow has called 'contact comfort.'

Consider the problem in terms of levels of psychological development, especially those of cognitive structure and object relationship. For the very young organism of any species, objects such as 'mother' do not exist in their own right but only as functional elements in the infant's economy which are assimilated in terms of the present only. When out of sight the object is out of mind, except perhaps as a fleeting image which may be recognized but which has no continuity, permanence, or substance. In Piaget's terms there is no 'conservation of the object'; in psychoanalytic terms there is no 'object constancy.' Distressing stimuli activate species characteristic behaviours, such as clinging, which will ordinarily be to the mother, who is there. For the infant this may represent 'contact comfort,' but its adaptive value in terms of survival is obvious, since the mother does in fact deal with all the dangers that in any way threaten the infant's existence. The infant may respond with clinging even if the distressing stimuli emanate from the object to which it clings since the infant's cognitive structure does not allow recognition of the sameness of the object. This may explain the findings of Rosenblum and Harlow (1963), i.e., the infants they studied did not recognize that the aversive stimuli were 'coming from mother.' We do not know yet if, or when, macaque infants growing up with their natural mothers achieve the cognitive structure necessary for object constancy and true object relationship to develop, as happens in the human infant when objects become detached from action, take on an independent and separate existence, and are endowed as such with emotional value. We know from the human that after object relationship has been established in the infant, intermittent maternal rejection, moderate and specific, plays a powerful role in further development, helping to establish modes of behaviour and systems of value. This is done by threatening the relationship, which the growing child must preserve, a task made more difficult by the fact that her rejection also provokes his aggressiveness to her. He responds by being good, by suppressing his aggressiveness, by behaving as she wants, and by seeking reassurance from her, as in clinging to her to prove that she still exists, and that she loves and accepts him. This is very different from the automatic clinging of the neonate despite the apparent similarities. Later, through processes of internalization and identification, and the emergence of superego functions, the complexity continues to grow, both behaviourally and intrapsychically.

For the monkey we can speak only of what we see, that maternal rejection increases the infant's efforts at attachment.

Another point to make is a simple fact we all know but should not overlook. Whatever the role of rejection, the *main* determinant of attachment is the quality, quantity, and variety of positive, mainly low-key, harmonious interactions between mother and infant, supporting the infant's physiological systems and building his psychosocial ones (Schneirla, 1959; Spitz, 1965).

With respect to the role of maternal rejection, here is one final comment of a rather speculative nature. In suggesting that rejection by the mother leads to increased strength of attachment in the young I appear to be in a dilemma, since Professor Hinde's data do show us compellingly that the more rejected infants do in fact spend more time *off* the mother, and since we all know that episodic maternal rejection is indeed a universal phenomenon as the young mature. Its very ubiquitousness may lead to a resolution of the dilemma. I would suggest that the function of maternal rejection is to be found in its biosocial significance. Rejection increases the tendency to attachment, primarily built on the basis described above, at the same time as it progressively denies the person of the mother as the object for attachment, thus leading to major attachments to *other* objects, an essential requirement of advanced societal living. Without dwelling on the further ramifications of this hypothesis, it may be noted that it tends to close the gap between Professor Hinde's position and mine — a gap which may be more apparent than real anyway.

Although we have worked with different species, under somewhat different conditions, and have analysed our data somewhat differently, yet, in many ways, the concordance of our data is more striking than the differences.

Essentially we differ only in our assessment of the way in which maternal rejection acts developmentally, his view being that it acts to increase the infant's independence, and my view being, in its simplest statement, that, within limits, rejection increases attachment. Actually, I believe that his own data support my view. He consistently finds, both in normal development and in relation to separation, that the frequency of maternal rejection correlates strongly with efforts by the infant to come closer to mother. This also helps us to understand his findings with respect to mother-loss. The more attached to the mother the infant is, the more distressed is he by her absence. This is quite consistent with studies by Fleener and Cairns (1970) of separation reactions in several non-primate mammals. They say 'Young lambs or dogs, after having been continuously housed with another animal, show considerable behavioural disturbance and vocal activity on being separated from their cohabitant. The extent of the disruption ... is significantly correlated with the tendency of the young animal to approach and remain with his cohabitant.' One can understand Professor Hinde's findings to indicate that, other considerations aside, the more the mother rejects the infant, the more dependent does the infant become, as manifested by greater efforts to approach her, and the more dependent he is on her, the more distressed is he by losing her. Put another way, we may say that the more inaccessible she is the greater is his effort to teach her, or perhaps his *need* to. In that sense, the loss of mother is the ultimate degree of inaccessibility, and we may expect from the infant the ultimate effort based on a markedly increased need. I would like to consider that need and effort and what happens to them.

It is noted above that the observed effects of mother-loss depend in part on *when* one looks. There is considerable evidence that there are *stages* to the reaction. Spitz (1946), who first described the serious effects of separation from mother in human infants, noted an initial apprehension and weepiness, followed by depression. If the mothers returned within a few months the infants recovered fully. If they did not return the infants developed what he called the 'hospitalism syndrome' — massive failure of physical and mental development, frequent illness, marasmus, cachexia, and often, early death (Spitz, 1945). Bowlby (1960) described *three* stages in *older* children — protest, despair, and detachment. Studies in monkeys by Harlow, Seay, and Hansen (1962, 1965), and by Professor Hinde himself (1966), reported initial protest, then despair. Heinicke and Westheimer (1965), in a detailed study of 2 – 3-year-old children in a residential nursery described *five* phases of psychic reaction which they saw as 'successive efforts at adaptation.'

There are some additional interesting things about our studies of pigtails and bonnets who had their mothers removed for four weeks (Kaufman and Rosenblum, 1967a, 1967b). The *initial* reaction in all was one of extreme

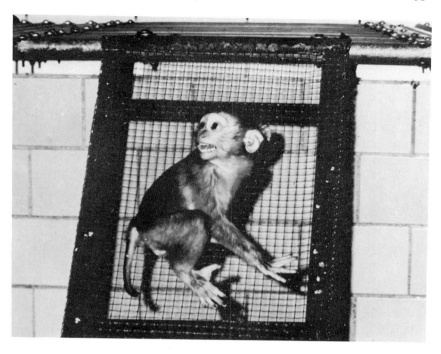

FIGURE 9   Agitated pigtail infant fleeing from rebuff by adult female he had approached. Note fear grimace while screaming. (From I.C. Kaufman and L.A. Rosenblum, The reaction to separation in infant monkeys: anaclitic depression and conservation-withdrawal. *Psychosom. Med.* 29 (1967), 648-75)

agitation with screaming, distress calls, pacing, searching head movements, frequent trips to the door and window, and movements towards other group members (Figure 9). In most pigtails studied this reaction persisted for about a day, during which time the infant neither ate nor slept; but the next day the infant showed a *severe depression*, sitting hunched over, almost rolled into a ball with the head often between the knees (Figure 10). When the face could be seen it had the appearance of dejection and sadness Darwin described and believed 'to be universally and instantly recognized as that of grief' (Figure 11). The infant became very inactive, did not play, and seemed disengaged from his environment (Figure 12). After five to six days of persistent depression the reaction began to lift with gradual re-engagement of, first, the inanimate environment, and then, of peers. By the end of the four weeks of separation the infant appeared fairly normal in his behaviour. In these pigtails, then, during the mother's absence, there were three successive stages —

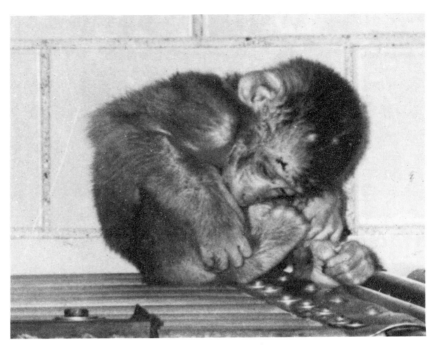

FIGURE 10 Depressed pigtail infant showing characteristic posture, including head between legs. Note slightly opened eyes as he sucks his penis. (From I.C. Kaufman and L.A. Rosenblum, The reaction to separation in infant monkeys: anaclitic depression and conservation-withdrawal. *Psychosom. Med.* 29 (1967), 648-75)

agitation, depression, and finally recovery. When the mother was returned there was an intense reunion, and all indices of mother/infant closeness remained high for three months. One pigtail infant did not show depression after the initial agitation. She managed to achieve considerable ventral contact and positive social interaction with other group adults, unlike the other infants who were rebuffed, whereupon she then entered the recovery phase. The interaction with other adults apparently was comfort-producing and allowed her to remain engaged with her environment.

We have also carried out comparable separations in bonnet infants. All showed *initial agitation* but none became depressed. All achieved as much ventral contact with other adults as they had had with their mothers. In effect they were adopted — held, and even nursed. One female with her own infant adopted and nursed two separated infants (Figure 13). Without question it was the overwhelming increase in interaction with other adults that characterized the reaction of the bonnet infants to separation, and that

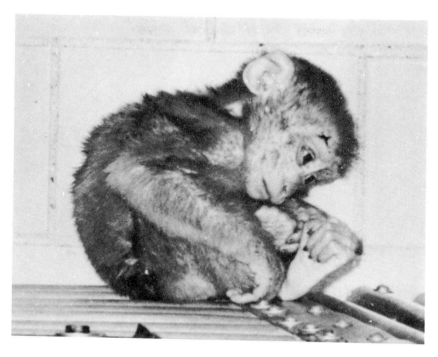

FIGURE 11   Depressed pigtail infant showing characteristic posture and dejected facies. (From I.C. Kaufman and L.A. Rosenblum, The reaction to separation in infant monkeys: anaclitic depression and conservation-withdrawal. *Psychosom. Med.* 29 (1967), 648-75)

seemed to provide quite adequate substitution for mother, so that the reaction was terminated after the first stage.

In the pigtail it is probable that the three stages are successive efforts at adaptation to the loss of mother. Distress calls were quite frequent in the *first* stage. In the wild, were the infant to become separated from the mother, the calls would surely have the effect of bringing her back, were she able. The monkey infants also showed restless pacing and searching which, in the wild, would be over a wider area and most likely would assist in reuniting the infant with his mother. However, this calling, searching reaction is not the kind of mechanism that can go on indefinitely, for at least two reasons. First of all, the increased movement and vocalization increase the risk of provoking aggression, either from conspecifics or from predators. Secondly, the markedly heightened activity is exhausting. Thus, we find that the agitated distress reaction comes to an end after a relatively short period of time.

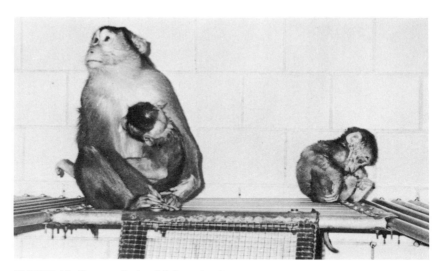

FIGURE 12 Depressed pigtail infant showing characteristic hunched-over posture with flexion throughout. He is completely disengaged from mother and infant nearby in ventral-ventral contact. (From I.C. Kaufman and L.A. Rosenblum, The reaction to separation in infant monkeys: anaclitic depression and conservation-withdrawal. *Psychosom. Med.* 29 (1967), 648-75)

The *second* stage we have described as a severe depression. There appears to be survival value in this also. First of all, there is an obvious conservation of energy and resources, achieved through the marked inactivity, and the posture which likely cuts down heat loss by reducing the exposed body surface. The posture also makes the infant literally smaller so that he presents less of a visual stimulus to other animals. The paucity and extreme slowness of movement also minimize notice of him by others. He is thus less likely to provoke aggression. Furthermore, the posture would reduce exposure to adverse elements – e.g., wind and rain.

Just as the stage-one reaction has time-limited survival value, the depressive reaction, if it continued unabated and indefinitely, would have a host of deleterious effects. This state of minimal action and interaction sharply curtails experience of the outside world, and would virtually bring further development to an end. The animal growing physically larger but otherwise not acquiring the personal and social skills of his species would not long survive, or would survive only as an outcast with no possibility of reproductive success.

The consequences of prolongation of this depressive reaction were tragically evident in the babies with the hospitalism syndrome described by Spitz

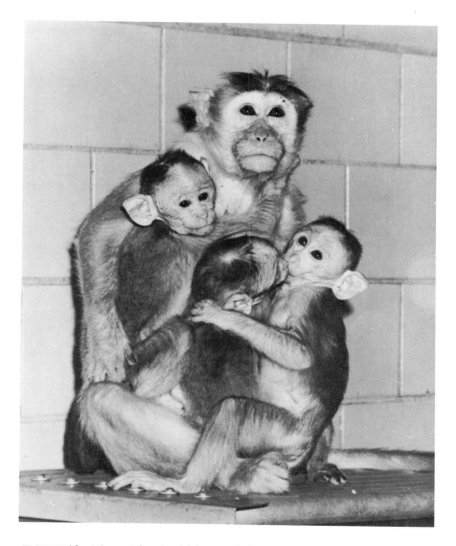

FIGURE 13 A bonnet female with her own infant and two separated infants whom she adopted. She nursed, carried, and protected these two infants throughout their separation

(1945). Not only did further development cease, but there was regression and ultimately no fitness for survival. This illustrates the fact that in the human, evolutionary adaptation has accentuated the role of the mothering figure to an exquisite degree. The human infant cannot survive without a mother. The monkey infant, on the other hand, from an early age, *is* able to survive without mother, and this was illustrated by the *third* stage of reaction: the recovery from the depression. This, we believe, he was able to do because of his locomotor ability. As Spitz noted, the human infant for a long time has no locomotor ability, and even when he begins to acquire it, he is very much dependent on other figures in the environment to provide the opportunities to use it. The monkey infant, however, after the first few weeks of life is able to move about, and within a relatively short time he has very considerable locomotor ability. This provides the mechanism which enables him on his own to re-engage the environment and to find new sources of comfort, with a reasonable likelihood of success, not only in surviving, but also in resuming development, acquiring new knowledge and new skills, and achieving social growth through interaction with peers and adults.

HUMAN COMPARISONS

Professor Hinde, in pointing out the similarity in response between bereft monkeys and humans, warned us that 'If the symptoms are similar in man and prelinguistic monkey, this in itself may place limits on the complexity of the explanatory hypothesis necessary in the human case' (p. 45). Of course he is right.

In comparing the reaction in monkeys with that in humans, it is necessary to consider developmental levels. The striking similarities of response, consisting of a sequence of agitated searching followed by a depressive reaction, suggest that the mediating mechanisms must be relatively undifferentiated biological response systems which are essentially common to these species.

In a theoretical paper, Frank (1954) offered 'the thesis that depression-elation responses constitute part of the inherent adaptive machinery available to the individual. They are employed automatically, unconsciously, and directly as adaptive measures under conditions when either in actuality or fantasy a relatively helpless individual is threatened with the loss of suitable care, protection, and sustenance.'

Engel and Reichsman (1956), in their classical study of the child Monica, described how she would withdraw in the presence of a stranger and even go to sleep, while showing profound reduction in the secretion of hydrochloric acid by the stomach. Drawing upon Frank's thesis, they labelled Monica's response as 'depression-withdrawal'; 'depression' because of 'the impact on the observer of the facial expression, posture, and inactivity, all of which call to mind a mood of dejection, sadness or depression'; and 'withdrawal' because of 'the turning away, the closing of the eyes, and the eventual sleep. The immobility and hypotonia may be seen as part of the withdrawal pattern as well as part of the affect disturbance.'

In subsequent publications Engel (1962) has elaborated this thesis further. Incorporating observations on infants and young children and the theorizing of Bibring (1953), he wrote, 'When we couple such observations with the recognition of the fact that even the most intense crying fit eventually terminates and the infant becomes quiescent, falls asleep, or even becomes comatose, even though the underlying needs have not been fulfilled, we are drawn to the conclusion that the central nervous system is organized to mediate two opposite patterns of response to a mounting need ... The first, broadly subsumed under the heading of flight-fight, involves activity, energy expenditure and engagement with the environment to control sources of supply and avert danger. The second, conservation-withdrawal, involves inactivity, energy conservation, raising of the stimulus barrier, and withdrawal from the environment. Each of these is seen as an inborn system, each with its own underlying mediating neural organization. The conservation-withdrawal system is a second biological defence organization which comes into play if and when the energy expenditures of the first (flight-fight) reaction threaten the organism with exhaustion before supplies are secured ...' He considers the first system to be the biological anlage of anxiety and the second of depression-withdrawal, these being in his view the two primary affects of unpleasure.

The monkey and human data, showing agitation, then depression, in response to the continued absence of mother or an adequate substitute, seem strongly to corroborate Engel's theory about the stages of biological response to a mounting need, based on available response systems. Support also comes from Mason's (1968) studies of hormonal system responses in avoidance conditioning. He found a two-stage sequence in which the initial response was by catabolic hormones, followed later by an outpouring of anabolic hormones. There is also recent neurophysiological evidence that the vertebrate nervous system is organized to subsume a comfort-distress dichotomy of whole organism reactions, each of which may appear in either a facilitated or suppressed form (Riss and Scalia, 1967).

The two responses described by Engel are both distress reactions, the first being associated with facilitation and the second with suppression. Facilitated distress is the reaction which tends to overcome or escape from the source of distress, or find again the source of comfort. Persistence of this high-energy catabolic disturbance is assumed to lead to changes in the internal milieu (probably chemical) that are essentially similar to the malaise of physical illness, and which induce through the diencephalic level a change in the adjustment from facilitation to suppression of the distress reaction. A collapsed posture, immobility, and a break with the environment ensue. This state of enforced rest, as in the physically sick organism, is the reaction which ordinarily permits subsequent recovery and survival.

From our earlier discussion we would say that the mother's absence provokes the distress reaction. The stages appear to represent successive efforts at adaptation based on available response systems, evolved for their selective advantage. Early in life these are common to monkey and man, so that we can understand the remarkable similarity between monkey and human infants in their reaction to separation. However, older children already show a more complicated reaction, and in adult humans the complexity is enormous, so that we must undo massive symbolic transformations to try to perceive the similarities.

Engel has described two stages of response to a mounting need, and our data support that. He also said that the affects involved in each stage are the biological anlage of anxiety and depression. This is convincing, but to a large extent it is clinical intuition. It is based in part on the phenomenological similarity but more on the affective states produced in us, the observers. We should not underestimate the importance of communicated affect, both in terms of its survival value and its role in social organization. The affect during agitation I would consider as undifferentiated apprehension, based on the infant experiencing uncertain incongruity as he matches his established plans of behaviour against the distressing environment – a precursor of anxiety. The affect during conservation-withdrawal I would consider as undifferentiated pessismism, based on unmanageable incongruity – the precursor of depression.

With experience, maturation, and learning a variety of changes occurs which leads to gross alterations in the response patterns. 'Mother' becomes a true object. Repertoires of behaviours and plans emerge, providing new coping and controlling mechanisms, including differentiation of the affects and their utilization as internal communicative signals. In both monkeys and humans, however, we may see in the young infant separated from mother the relatively undifferentiated biopsychological response patterns.

There is of course much more that one could say about the later significance in the human of object loss and its relation to separation anxiety, stranger anxiety, the development of the ego and superego, and psychosomatic illness, to mention but a few. However, I shall conclude by expressing my thanks to Professor Hinde for telling us about his very important studies and stimulating me to attempt further clarification in my own mind of an area of study with which I have been preoccupied for many years.

PETER MARLER

3   Constraints on Learning:
Development of Bird Song*

Recent work on the structure of language and on the early attempts of children to speak has led to a revolution in our thinking about the requirements for the development of language (Chomsky, 1967; Lenneberg, 1967). Instead of thinking of the child as completely dependent on his parents for everything that emerges in language behaviour, a view which regards the child as though it were a blank slate on which experience can write almost anything, the child is thought of as having a more positive, interactive role, selective in its learning, imposing its own kind of order on the stimulation received in speech of parents and siblings. The basic issue here has significance beyond language development, to learning in general. The role of predispositions that organisms bring to tasks of learning has been neglected for too long.

Such predispositions can take many forms, and it would need an entire book to survey them all. During the last ten years, my colleagues and I have been studying the role of learning in the development of birdsong. This review of some of the results is intended to demonstrate the role of predispositions in birdsong learning. Further, if brought into relief, this illustrates some of the ways in which the study of learning, as it takes place under natural conditions, highlights deficiencies in the old behaviouristic notion of the *tabula rasa*.

Learning plays an important role in the ontogeny of several aspects of communicative behaviour. In many animals learning is undoubtedly important in the development of responsiveness to signals. The use to which signals are put in nature cannot be understood without appreciating this basic role that learning plays. But the modification by learning of the behaviour that generates signals per se is more rarely found within the animal kingdom. The dependence of many song birds on learning in the development of their vocalizations is thus unusual.

* The research described in this report was supported by grants from the National Science Foundation (GB-16606) and the National Institutes of Mental Health (MH-14651)

One might think that the first place to look for evidence of vocal learning would be other primates than ourselves. To date, a non-human primate with any facility in vocal imitation has yet to be discovered. There have been some laboratory studies, notably those of Hayes and Hayes who raised the young female chimpanzee Vicki in their home with the aim of, among other things, teaching her to speak (Hayes, 1951). They were able to get her to utter three words well, 'papa,' 'mama,' and 'cup.' The results are very interesting, but a survey of the methods they were compelled to use in order to bring these three words into Vicki's repertoire makes it clear that they were dealing with something quite different from the capacity for free vocal imitation, as this is manifest in the speech development of children. As Kellogg (1968) has expressed it in a review of this work, their most important finding was 'the discovery that the sound patterns were extremely hard for the ape to master, that they never came naturally or easily, and that she had trouble afterwards in keeping the patterns straight.' If you press the search for other organisms with a facility for vocal imitation comparable to that of man, with the possible exception of dolphins, the only other well-documented cases come from birds.

The capacity of some birds to imitate human speech is well-known, and there are some psychologists who feel that study of this capacity might somehow illuminate our understanding of speech development. I can perhaps best express my disagreement with this view by asking whether a student of speech development in children, seeking to learn whether the child brings any special predispositions to the task, would find it instructive to try to teach the child sounds of any other species. If predispositions exist, they are likely to be species specific and thus will be most clearly manifest within the framework of the patterns of behaviour which the species itself generates. It is almost as odd to try to teach a bird speech as it would be to teach a child birdsong. The result might be of interest, but the extent to which it would illuminate normal vocal development is questionable. Rather we should seek an understanding of the role which learning plays in vocal development as it occurs under natural conditions. Approached in this way, it may be that a comparison between organisms as remote as a bird and a human child may perhaps elucidate our understanding of the human case, at least at the conceptual level.

In what follows, it is suggested that we can discern parallels between the development of song in a bird like the white-crowned sparrow, which we have studied at some length, and some of the more elementary properties of speech development. In each case, learning plays a major role in the development of the adult morphology of the vocalizations. In both birds and man, local dialects are a consequence of this dependence upon learning. In each we can see some evidence that the ability for vocal learning reaches a peak at a certain age.

In birds, and perhaps in man too, there is reason to think of hearing as having two roles, both important for development of song or speech. On the one hand is the capacity to hear environmental sounds. On the other is the more subtle capacity to hear one's own voice. There is some reason to think that the kinds of reinforcement that underlie vocal learning may perhaps be similar in the avian and human case. Finally, there even seems to be a parallel in the properties of the physiological machinery which underlies learned vocalization. This is a phenomenon discovered recently by Dr Fernando Nottebohm (1970a, 1970b). He has evidence of lateralization in the neural control of vocal performance in birds, reminiscent of the cerebral dominance of speech control in man.

The white-crowned sparrow was selected for many of these studies because we have found that there are dialects in its natural song. 'Dialects,' in this sense, are consistent differences in the morphology of vocalizations in populations of the same bird species which are separate but living close together, too close to tempt one to attribute the difference to genetic causes (Figure 1).

If a young male white-crowned sparrow is raised in isolation from four to five days of age in the laboratory, he will subsequently develop a song with certain normal characteristics – the duration and tonal quality of these sounds will match those of wild birds. But the detail will be quite unlike that of any song recorded from a wild male white-crowned sparrow (Figure 2). In order to restore normal development in such an individual in the laboratory, it suffices to play a recorded natural song to him, perhaps sixty times a day for three weeks, somewhere roughly between the tenth and fiftieth days of age. Given such exposure, he will, some months hence, as he becomes sexually mature, begin to sing on normal schedule, quickly approximating an imitation of the model to which he was exposed several months earlier. He will approximate it in two senses. The song he produces will be a natural one, now falling within the class of patterns to be described from wild white-crowned sparrows. But in addition, he will produce a detailed imitation of the particular dialect to which he was exposed during that critical period. Exposure later than about fifty days of age has little or no effect (Marler, 1970) (Figure 3).

Here then we see the first constraint on song learning: the limitation of this ability to a particular period of life. Further experimentation reveals constraints of another kind. Suppose that we present the young male bird within its acoustical chamber with a choice of what he will imitate. Instead of giving playback on his own species song alone, we alternate recordings of his own species with that of another. The learning is selective. Even though the

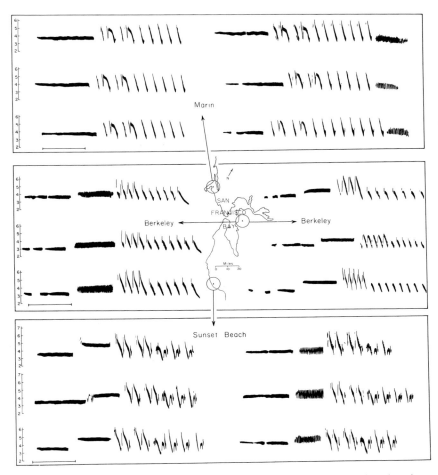

FIGURE 1   Dialects in song of the male white-crowned sparrow. Birds at three locations in California, in the San Francisco Bay area, have distinctly different song patterns. The dialect is especially evident in the fine structure of the second part of each song. Sound spectrograms of six birds are shown from each area. The frequency scale is marked in kHz, and 0.5 second time markers are provided (from Marler, 1970)

young male is incapable of generating a natural white-crowned sparrow song without access to a model, he seems to possess an ability to recognize the appropriate model for imitation. Thus he will, for example, reject the song of a close relative such as the song sparrow. If he is presented only with the song of this species during the critical period, he will reject it, and develop song as though he had had no exposure at all.

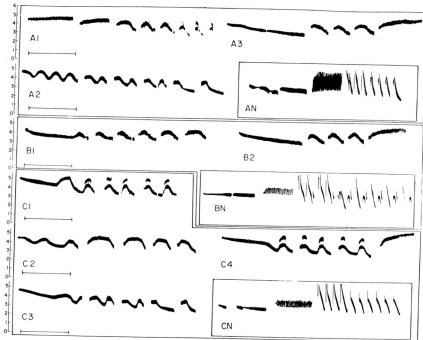

FIGURE 2 Songs of nine male white-crowned sparrows reared together in a large sound-proof room from an age of 5-8 days. They were taken from three different areas and the sound spectrograms are boxed with a sample of the dialect of each home area (AN, BN, and CN). Scales as in Figure 1 (from Marler, 1970)

Reflecting on much of the work on animal and human learning, this seems to be a point that we are prone to overlook. In many situations, perhaps all, there must be some constraints on learning. Some appreciation of the natural history of learning would make the evolution of such constraints seem almost inevitable, which is perhaps what Konrad Lorenz had in mind with his conception of the 'innate schoolmarm.' If you stand by the nest of a white-crowned sparrow and listen, the singing bird closest to you is just as likely to be a male song sparrow as a white-crowned sparrow. It would thus be hazardous if the young male were completely open to all kinds of auditory input in this situation.

This guidance of learning in the male sparrow is reminiscent in a very general sense of what Chomsky and Lenneberg tell us about language development in children — that they could not generate a language with all of its underlying grammar if they were totally dependent on the input received from speech that they hear. We are told that, at the level of deep structure, all

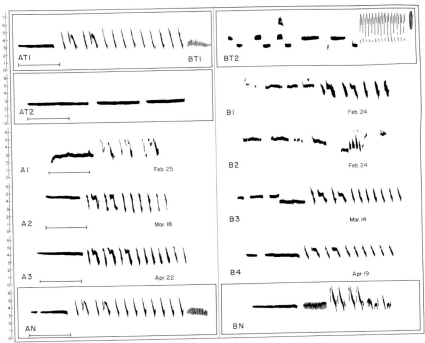

FIGURE 3 The development of song in two isolated male white-crowned sparrows (A1-3 and B1-4), trained in youth for 21 days with a recording of normal song (AT1). A song of another species was also presented, Harris' sparrow, *Zonotrichia querula* for bird A (35-56 days); song sparrow, *Melospiza melodia*, for bird B (8-28 days). Only the conspecific song was imitated (see A3 and B4). Scales as in Figure 1 (from Marler, 1970)

languages have essentially the same kind of syntax. This would be very unlikely if human societies had no underlying guidelines or constraints on language development.

Here, as with other aspects of our behaviour, we are liable to forget that the capacity for modifying behaviour through learning, invaluable in the right circumstances, can also be harmful when operating without guidelines, in the wrong situations, or used in inappropriate ways. Superstitions in man and animals are cases in point.

If any species relies upon a complex set of learned traits as the fundaments upon which its social behaviour and ecology are constructed, it would be very surprising if the direction in which learning most readily occurs in generating these patterns of behaviour should be left completely to chance. Language is the pedestal on which much of our own biology is based, and just as it makes sense that song learning is guided by a set of constraints, it is perhaps not too much of an extrapolation to think of guidance in the kind of grammatical structure that a child can most readily generate as valuable to human survival.

We have noted that various lines of evidence point to the existence of constraints imposed on the process of song learning, both in time, such that there are critical periods when learning takes place most readily, and in the acoustical patterns which are most readily learned. In some species, there are also social constraints involved. However, in the white-crowned sparrow and the chaffinch the restrictions on the type of sound that will be learned are not attributable to social influences, since they are manifest in a bird raised in isolation from a few days after birth, with selection made from sounds coming through a loudspeaker. In these cases the constraints must be in some sense endogenous to the organism. Two rather different kinds of endogenous mechanisms might impose conspecific constraints on the learning process.

One possibility is that motor guidance could be provided — by the structure of the sound-producing equipment, in this case the respiratory machinery. The syrinx and its associated membranes, muscles and resonators must impose some restrictions on what sounds can be produced. Could these restrictions be sufficiently specific to provide a basis for selection of conspecific song for imitation, and rejection of the songs of close relatives?

There are several reasons for doubting that such motor constraints would be sufficient. The sound-producing equipment will of course set limits, but the evidence suggests that these limits are very broad. No difference has been detected between the syringes of closely related birds such as the white-crowned sparrow and the song sparrow. The structure of the bird syrinx is in fact known to be a conservative trait that changes only slowly in the course of evolution. It is widely used as a taxonomic character at the higher levels of phylogenetical classification. There are many examples of species with similar syringeal structure producing very different vocalizations. Thus a chaffinch and a bullfinch have similar syringes, but a bullfinch raised by hand and imprinted on its human keeper will imitate a great variety of unnatural sounds, including tunes on the flageolet (Thorpe, 1955). A chaffinch, like a white-crowned sparrow, is very restricted in what it will imitate (Thorpe, 1961).

If a white-crowned sparrow is deafened early in life, it develops a song more abnormal than that of an intact bird raised in isolation. The few normal song characteristics that the social isolate develops are lost if the bird cannot hear its own voice (Konishi, 1965) (Figure 4). This discovery has led to the invocation of a sensory mechanism to guide vocal development. The hypothesis has gradually developed over a period of years that certain song birds

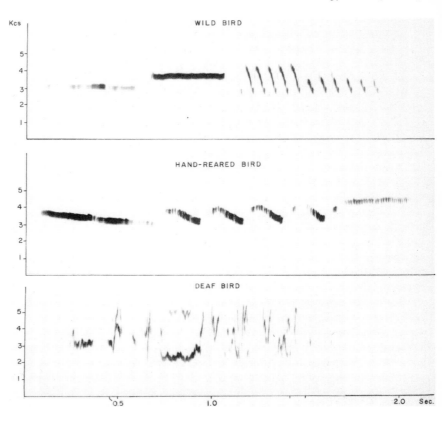

FIGURE 4   Songs of three male white-crowned sparrows, one a wild bird, one raised by hand in isolation from normal song, and one deafened in youth (from Konishi, 1965)

develop vocalizations by reference to something we may think of as an 'auditory template' (Marler, 1963; Konishi, 1965; Konishi and Nottebohm, 1969; Marler, 1970). This template is visualized as a mechanism or mechanisms residing at one or more locations in the auditory pathway, providing a model to which the bird can match its vocalizations. Accomplishment of this matching is presumed to take place over a period of time, as the bird acquires sufficient skill in the control of its sound-producing equipment to generate eventually a perfect match with the dictates of the template.

In some species, such as the song sparrow, an individual raised in complete isolation from species members seems to possess a sufficiently well specified template that it can generate normal song, as long as it can hear itself (Mulligan, 1966). However, in other species, such as the white-crowned

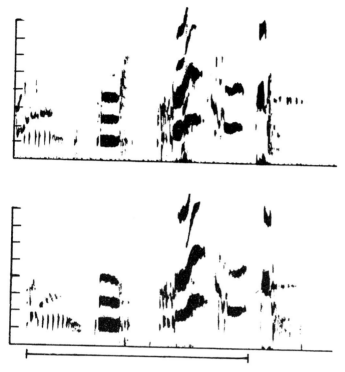

FIGURE 5 Song of a male Bengalese finch (above) used as a foster parent to a male Zebra finch (below). The Zebra finch learned the song of his foster father. Scales as in Figure 1, time marker 0.5 seconds (from Immelmann, 1969)

sparrow or the chaffinch, the initial specifications for the template are less complete.

A male white-crowned sparrow raised in social isolation from a week or so of age will develop a song which, although abnormal in its over-all pattern, does nevertheless possess certain natural characteristics, particularly the sustained pure tones which are one basic element in the natural song. These pure tones are largely absent from the song of a bird deafened early in life. Thus a male white-crowned sparrow already seems to possess at the age of 10-50 days a crude auditory template of the song. Although this does not suffice to generate normal song by itself, it may be adequate to focus the young male's attention on sounds of his own species rather than those of others to be heard in the same area such as the song sparrow. We presume that, as he listens to conspecific song, the properties are somehow incorporated in the template, which thus becomes more highly specified, embodying properties both of the species song in general, and of the particular local dialect which the male has experienced. When the male subsequently comes into song, this more refined template will now guide development along a normal pathway, as long as he can hear his own voice.

The essential notion exemplified by this 'template' is that of active filtering of incoming sensory information, not unrelated to what is implied by von Uexküll's 'innate schema' and by Lorenz's 'innate release mechanism' (Lorenz, 1951). The same template can serve both as a kind of filter for focusing attention on sounds that match its crude specification, and as a vehicle for retaining information about the more detailed characteristics of sound learned, and subsequently translating it into vocal activity.

Although social restrictions on the direction taken by song learning can be dispensed with in the chaffinch and the white-crowned sparrow, they are critically important in some other species. Nicolai (1959) has evidence that young bullfinches selectively learn both the song and one of the other vocalizations from their father. He discovered this when a male bullfinch raised by canaries learned some canary phrases and in turn transmitted them to his offspring. Similarly the sons of a male bullfinch that had been raised by hand and taught to whistle a tune learned their father's abnormal song from him, even though normal songs could be heard nearby. Young zebra finches will show a preference for learning the songs of the father, or of a foster father of another species (Figure 5), even though they will select conspecific song when given an even choice (Immelmann, 1969).

No doubt song learning is guided along social channels in other bird species which have bonds between parent and young that persist through the period during which learning takes place. However such bonds are of only brief duration in many small birds, as in the chaffinch and the white-crowned sparrow whose families break up as the young are weaned. Thus these species require some other mechanism for ensuring the selectivity of song learning.

What is the reinforcement or reward in vocal learning? In his autism theory of language learning, Mowrer (1950, 1958) proposed that each sound acquires secondary reinforcing properties as a result of association with primary reinforcement of other kinds from the parent — pleasurable sensation, approbation, and so on. A similar process may underlie song learning in species in which social constraints are operating to impose selectivity on the learning. Since many song birds feed their young by mouth, it is not inconceivable that direct reinforcement by parental feeding might be involved in some species (Mundinger, 1969). Alternatively some other kind of parental stimulation, perhaps given in response to utterance of similar sounds by the young, might serve as a reinforcement (Figure 6).

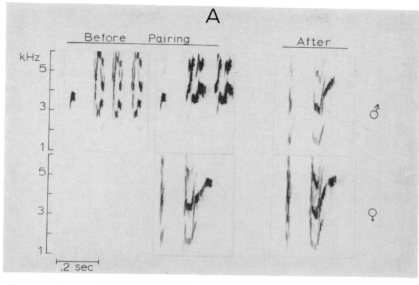

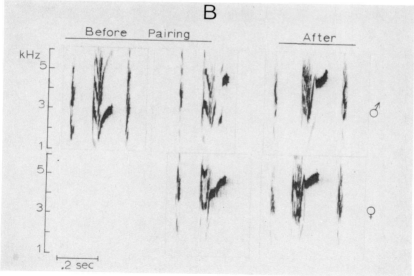

FIGURE 6 Flight calls of two pairs of siskins, *Carduelis spinus*, recorded before and after pairing. Both pairs converged on common patterns after males and females were put together. Pairs engage in courtship feeding and this case of vocal learning could conceivably be associated with food reinforcement (from Mundinger, 1970)

One gathers that some investigators are sceptical of the adequacy of Mowrer's autism theory as a complete explanation of speech learning in children. Even with talking birds, where Mowrer felt this hypothesis to be especially relevant, Foss (1964) found that mynah birds learned a whistle sound played through a loudspeaker just as well without simultaneous food reinforcement as with it, there being no social stimulation in either case.

Neither direct nor indirect social stimulation can be invoked to explain song learning in the white-crowned sparrow. In the first place, the initial phase of learning precedes utterance of copies of the sounds heard by a period of many weeks. In the second, training is accomplished effectively by presenting recorded sounds through a loudspeaker, with no other concomitant stimulation. In this species production of a sound resembling that heard previously during the critical period is in some sense an intrinsically reinforcing act.

We can discern many points in the process of song learning at which genetic influences might readily intrude. The structure of the sound-producing equipment – the syrinx and its associated resonators and respiratory apparatus – vary under the control of genetic factors. As in embryological development, variations in the timing of critical periods may be under genetic control. The same must be true of processes of reinforcement. Species differences in the structure of the so-called 'auditory template' might be under genetic control. The songs of early-deafened juncos, song sparrows, and white-crowned sparrows, are much more similar than their normal songs (Figure 7), which are radically different in many respects (Konishi, 1964, 1965; Mulligan, 1966; Marler and Mundinger, in press).

Thus, although there is ample evidence that some birds engage in vocal learning in the course of normal development, it is also clear that the capacity for learning is by no means unlimited. Rather it takes place within a set of constraints which seem designed to ensure that the learning bird's attention shall be focused on a set of sounds that is biologically relevant, guided by appropriate reinforcers, during a particular period of the life cycle.

The interplay between learning and the predispositions that the bird brings to the learning situation, here brought into rather sharp relief, is likely to be a widespread, even universal phenomenon in animal learning as it takes place under natural conditions. Konrad Lorenz (1965) feels it to be 'an inescapable logical necessity to assume that learning, like any other organic function regularly achieving survival value, is performed by organic structures evolved in the course of phylogeny under the selection pressure of just that survival value.'

We must consider the possibility that human learning is subject to such constraints as well. It is indicated above that some of the elementary guidelines for human speech development may bear a formal resemblance to the

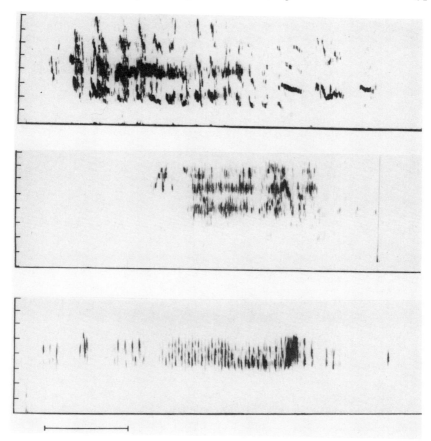

FIGURE 7 Songs of males of three species all deafened early in life. Top: Oregon junco, *Junco oreganus*. Middle: white-crowned sparrow, *Zonotrichia leucophrys*. Bottom: song sparrow, *Melospiza melodia*. As can be determined from the original sources (Konishi, 1964, 1965; Mulligan, 1966), the songs of early-deafened birds are highly variable. These three were selected for their similarity. Songs of hearing individuals of these species are much more divergent. Scales as in Figure 1, time marker 0.5 seconds.

constraints on birdsong learning, even though the accomplishments eventually learned are on an altogether different plane of functional complexity. There is one more hint that the parallels may be more than trivial.

Physiologists have stated in print that the lateralization of cerebral control, as we see it in speech, is a human phenomenon. It was surprising and exciting when Dr Fernando Nottebohm (1970s, 1970b), doing experiments on the de-innervation of the syrinx of birds, discovered an apparent parallel. He took adult male chaffinches, already in full song, and exposed the syrinx at the base of the trachea. The syrinx receives symmetrical innervation from the two sides of the brain, mainly from the hypoglossus. After severing the innervation on one side, the bird recovered within a matter of hours, and he recorded the song then produced.

When he severed the innervation on the right side there were some slight deficits in the song – some of the simple syllables from which the song is constructed simply dropped out. By superimposing sound spectrograms of pre- and post-operative song, he found that the timing of the remaining elements is the same, but that certain elements have dropped out. Effects of the same operation on the left side, leaving the right side intact, were much more drastic. They were of two kinds, and it is not quite clear what underlies the alternatives. One was the complementary result to de-innervation on the right side: all of the complex syllables within the song dropped out to leave a very simple utterance, the remaining sounds again retaining their original timing. The other thing that sometimes happened was that instead of these complex syllables being totally lost, they were replaced by blasts of noise. Cutting the nerves to the right side thus resulted either in total loss of complex syllables or reversion to a very elementary kind of acoustical output. There was asymmetry in the control on right or left sides.

Repeating this with a number of birds Nottebohm established that in the male chaffinch the left side plays the dominant role. This is curiously reminiscent of the dominance of the left cerebral hemisphere in the control of speech in most people. There is another odd parallel: if this operation is performed, somewhat earlier in life, on a young male chaffinch who has yet to come into full song, the bird, given time to proceed through normal development, can generate typical song with the subordinate side. This is compellingly reminiscent of children who suffer early brain damage and who are then able to sustain normal speech with what would have been the subordinate hemisphere.

What do we make of such a comparison, if we are ready to entertain it at all? Obviously, it cannot be suggested that birds have language. In fact, it is obvious that birds are using this capacity for vocal learning in quite a different way from what early man must have done. Nevertheless, some aspects of the process of speech development and its neural control do not seem to be unique to man. At the very least, this kind of exercise in which we sift out species specific traits from those traits which are shared with other species may allow us to concentrate on those which are truly unique. Birds which learn their songs do not necessarily have a more complex social organization or ecology than birds in which learning does not play this important role. This serves as a reminder that in trying to retrace the evolution of early man, identification of the onset of the capacity for vocal learning would not, by itself, help very much. It is equally important to define the use to which the species is able to put this new capacity. This becomes as much a question of ecology and sociology as of ethology, psychology, and linguistics. Only by attending to the viewpoints of such diverse disciplines as these can the ethologist hope to make any lasting contribution to our understanding of the biology of man.

In return, the ethologist can offer some general positions that may be useful in approaching problems of human behaviour. The likelihood that organisms have evolved constraints that guide biologically important learning processes is perhaps germane to the ontogeny of human behaviour patterns, and especially to the development of language.

WILLIAM A. MASON, SUZANNE D. HILL,
CURTIS E. THOMSEN

4 Perceptual Aspects of Filial Attachment in Monkeys*

This article will approach the attachment of the infant rhesus monkey to an artificial mother as a problem for perceptual analysis. Monkeys come into the world equipped with a few highly organized and strongly motivated behaviours that permit them to make an effective initial adjustment to the mother. The infants are 'pre-programmed' to adapt to the maternal ecology: they can cling to the mother's body, locate the breast, seize the nipple and suck – and they can accomplish these acts with little or no maternal assistance.

Ordinarily, all these early filial responses are directed toward one and the same object – which is, of course, the mother – and the responses work together. It is possible, however, to break up this unifocal pattern by arranging the situation so that different filial responses are directed toward different objects. Thus, the animal could be provided with one object to cling to, and another to suckle from. This procedure was followed, in fact, in Harlow's early experiments in which artifical mothers were used to assess the relative contributions of clinging and nursing to the filial attachment. As one would expect, the animal learns under such circumstances to go to one object if it want to cling and to another if it wants to suckle (Harlow and Zimmermann, 1958).

But if it is possible to 'fragment' the mother by assigning different maternal functions to different objects, might it not also be possible that in natural circumstances the infant is going through the converse of this process – that he is, in fact, organizing diverse experiences with a single physical object to construct an integrated whole? Can we say that as the filial attachment develops, the infant is putting together the various attributes and functions experienced through different modalities to create a perceptual structure of the mother as a single multi-faceted entity? This seems reasonable in

* This research was supported by grants HD-03915 and FR-00164 from the US National Institutes of Health

principle, but how does such a synthesis actually come about? How can one trace the emergence of mother-as-object?

Fortunately, we know that the senses are not equivalent in the early development of the filial attachment in rhesus macaques, and we can use this fact to good advantage in setting up our approach. In Piaget's terms one could say that the newborn monkey is equipped with a maternal schema which is tuned chiefly to tactile information. Clearly this must change: as development proceeds this primitive tactile schema is extended and enriched by the assimilation of new information. Intuitively, this seems particularly obvious with respect to visual information, for in the beginning the infant macaque is almost completely indifferent to what its mother looks like, so long as she has the proper feel. It will cling with equal vigour to the body of its real mother, or to a towel, a diaper, or a rug. It seems to derive substantial emotional reassurance from the mere act of clinging to any of these objects. As vision comes into the picture, however, one assumes that the monkey becomes more discriminating and selective in its choice of maternal objects. It is eventually able to recognize its own specific 'mother' from a distance and from various angles of regard; it distinguishes her from other individuals; it seems to derive from the mere sight of her some of the same emotional benefits that at first only contact-clinging could provide. Until some such integration is achieved one might say that there is no perceptual or phenomenal object of attachment. The formation of an attachment to a specific maternal object thus implies that vision and touch are brought into a new working relationship. It is this developmental process that will concern us here.

We are investigating perceptual aspects of attachment in several different studies, most of which are still in progress. We have selected one experiment for discussion here in order to illustrate the general method of approach and the kind of results that may be anticipated.

The subjects are infant rhesus monkeys, separated from their mothers on the first day of life and housed individually in cages with a distinctive red-and-white checkered interior. Each cage (Figure 1) contains an artificial mother consisting of a simple 'body' (7 in. long, 4 in. wide, 1½ in. high) covered with blue-green acrylic fur. We have two rearing groups. One group ($N = 8$) has a clear plastic door at the front of the living cage which allows the animal to see other monkeys and the general nursery environment; the cages of the second group ($N = 10$) are completely enclosed. For the moment, however, we will treat all 18 animals as a single group. To save time we will limit the discussion to just one of the several measures of affect that we record – distress vocalizations, i.e., 'coos' and screams – and to one of our tests (see Mason, Hill, and Thomsen, forthcoming, for further details).

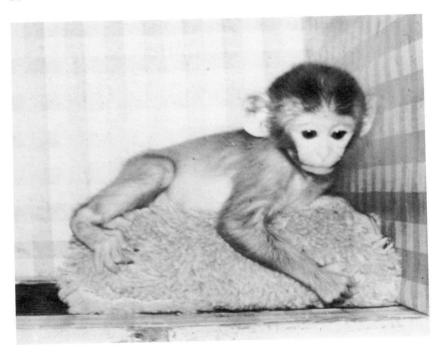

FIGURE 1   Living cage and the familiar artificial mother

In this test the monkey is observed in two different environments. One, the familiar environment (*FE*), simulates the dimensions and the red-and-white checkered interior of the living cage; the other, the unfamiliar environment (*UE*), is encountered only in the test situation. It has the same floor dimensions as the living cage, but has a higher ceiling, and the compartment is painted white, except for one wall which contains a variety of coloured patterns on a green background. The animal is observed in each of these test compartments while alone, or with the familiar surrogate or a stranger, both of which are available for clinging in some tests, and enclosed in a plastic box in others. In other words, in each environment we present five object conditions: (1) the familiar artificial mother accessible to vision and touch (*F*); (2) the familiar surrogate encased in clear plastic (*Ⓕ*); (3) the strange surrogate (*S*), accessible to vision and touch; (4) the strange surrogate encased in clear plastic (*Ⓢ*). The stranger is encountered only in the test situation. Its body is the same as the living cage surrogate, and it is covered with the same acrylic fur, but the fur is brown rather than blue-green; the

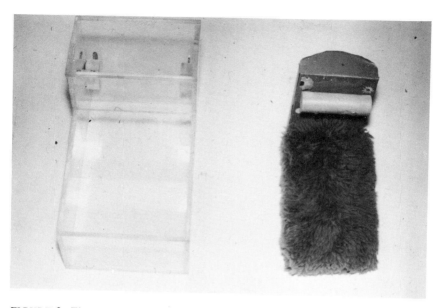

FIGURE 2 The strange artificial mother. On the left is the plastic box which contains the surrogate for the enclosed condition Ⓢ

unfamiliar surrogate also has a distinctive 'head' which the living cage surrogate lacks (Figure 2); (5) no object in the test environment (N).

Beginning at approximately two weeks of age and at monthly intervals thereafter, each monkey receives ten five-minute sessions in each of the ten possible test conditions (two environments, five conditions in each environment).

Let us consider first whether the various object conditions have reliable differential effects on distress vocalizations. From the data in Figure 3, which presents results for the first three months (phases) of testing, it is evident that they do. Differences among the five conditions are significant in both environments and in every phase of testing and the order of effectiveness shows no obvious changes across sessions ($p < 0.001$, Friedman).

These findings indicate that from the beginning of testing the monkeys distinguish among the various test conditions. But what can the results tell us about the roles of visual and tactual information as sources of emotional reassurance? This question has several different aspects that we can treat separately.

First, one might ask how vision compares with touch as a source of reassurance. Our results confirm fully the primacy of Harlow's 'contact

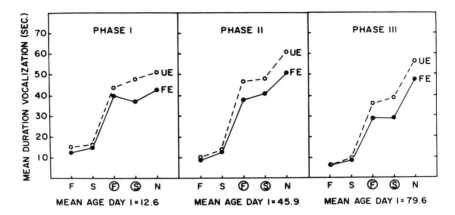

FIGURE 3 Mean duration of distress vocalizations in familiar *FE*) and unfamiliar (*UE*) environments. *F* = familiar artificial mother, totally accessible. *S* = strange artificial mother, totally accessible. Ⓕ= familiar artificial mother encased in clear plastic. ⒮= strange artificial mother encased in clear plastic. *N* = no object

comfort' during the first three months of life. Being able to cling to the visible surrogate is vastly more effective than visual access alone, and this is a true of the stranger as of the familiar surrogate. The differences are significant for both environments and in all test phases (*F* vs. Ⓕ, *S* vs. ⓈⓈ, *p*<0.01, Wilcoxon).

Even though unrestricted access to the surrogate is more effective than vision alone, it does not follow that visual information is without influence. The second question, then, is at what point in development does visual information modify emotional responsiveness? Our results indicate that visual familiarity has a definite effect from the very beginning of testing. Consider, for example, the effects of the test compartment. In all phases of testing the level of vocalization is significantly lower in the familiar environment than in the unfamiliar environment (*p*<0.05, Wilcoxon). The differences are present under all conditions, but they are largest when no claspable objects are present.

Another way of assessing the effects of visual familiarity is to compare the familiar surrogate with the stranger. Here, of course, we can consider the surrogates under the two conditions of availability — that it, unlimited access and visual access only. The results show that the familiar surrogate is more effective than the stranger, particularly when it can be contacted as well as seen. Under this condition differences are present from the first test phase, and they are statistically reliable in the last two phases (*p*<0.05, Wilcoxon). When both surrogates are encased in plastic there is again a suggestion that the familiar surrogate is more effective than the stranger, although the differences here are not reliable in any phase — at least as measures by vocalization. Our data on heart rate, however, show a reliable difference in response to the two shielded surrogates by phase II.

These results show that familiar visual input can be a significant source of emotional reassurance even in the first few weeks of life. But our test situation contains two different sources of familiar visual stimuli — one, an object that has been associated with clinging, and the other, the checkered interior of the living cage. The third question is, how do these two sources of familiar visual stimulation compare in effectiveness? The answer depends upon the phase of testing. The relevant comparison here is between the empty familiar environment (*FE, N*) and the enclosed familiar surrogate in the unfamiliar environment (*UE,* Ⓕ). The results are presented in Figure 4. In the first test phase there is little if any difference between these conditions. By phase II there is some suggestion that the familiar environment and the encased surrogate are no longer equivalent. Vocalizations are lower in the presence of the surrogate. Although the difference is not reliable in phase II, it becomes so in phase III ($p < 0.05$, Wilcoxon). It would thus appear that the encased familiar surrogate and the checkered interior of the living cage are about equally effective initially as sources of emotional reassurance, but that as development proceeds the artificial mother becomes more effective than the environment.

This outcome would be expected if one assumes that the intimate association between vision and clinging will enhance the visual effectiveness of the surrogate. But the matter does not appear to be quite as simple as this associational interpretation would suggest. Consider Figure 5, in which the enclosed surrogate stranger in the unfamiliar environment (*UE,* Ⓢ) is compared with the empty familiar environment (*FE, N*). In phase I, the shielded stranger in the novel environment is substantially *less* effective than the empty familiar environment ($p < 0.02$, Wilcoxon), which is precisely what one would expect. In the next two phases, however, the stranger is *more* effective, although not significantly so.

Thus, in spite of the vast difference in familiarity between the stranger and living cage surrogate, by the second month of life either of them in a plastic box in a novel environment is more effective in reducing vocalizations than the empty simulated living cage. Furthermore, the level of vocalizations in both environments is significantly lower in phases II and III when either of the encased surrogates is present than when the environments contain no objects.

How do we interpret these results? Are both enclosed surrogates becoming more effective as testing proceeds, or are the monkeys simply becoming more distressed by the empty test compartments? This might seem to be a pseudo-

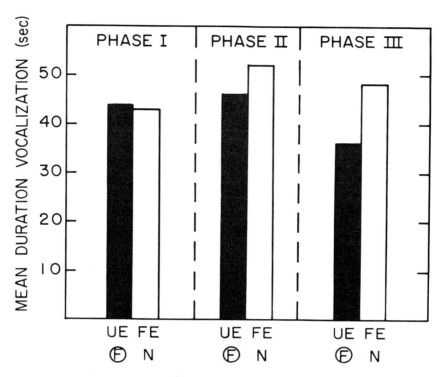

FIGURE 4 Mean duration of distress vocalizations in the presence of the encased familiar artificial mother in the unfamiliar environment (*UE*, Ⓕ) and in the empty familiar environment (*FE, N*)

question, but we believe that it can be answered. The answer is that the empty environment becomes more distressing. The evidence can be seen most clearly if one considers for each phase the percentage of total vocalizations attributable to each object condition. This is shown for the combined environments in Figure 6. Note that over phases the empty condition accounts for progressively more of the total amount of vocalizations ($p < 0.001$, Friedman). Although both surrogates encased in plastic account for a progressively smaller percentage of total vocalizations as the animals become older, the changes are small, they are non-significant, and the difference between the novel and familiar surrogates is essentially constant across phases. A second important developmental effect is suggested by this figure. When both surrogates are available for contact, the familiar surrogate shows a larger increase in effectiveness across phases than the stranger, although the direction of change is the same for both.

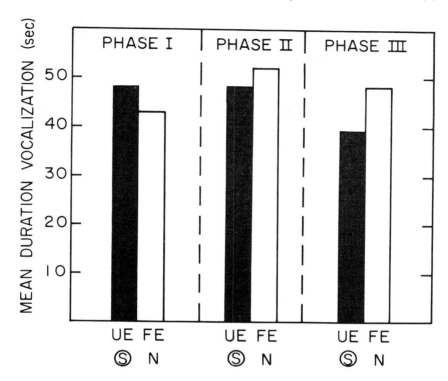

FIGURE 5 Mean duration of distress vocalizations in the presence of the encased stranger in the unfamiliar environment (*UE,* Ⓢ) and in the empty familiar environment (*FE, N*)

We might summarize these developmental changes as follows: in the first month of life the monkey's emotional reactions indicate a clear differentiation of claspable objects from all other conditions, but there is little difference in the response to familiar versus unfamiliar claspable objects, or to non-claspable objects versus the empty test compartments. Nevertheless, visual familiarity must be considered an effective source of emotional reassurance even at this early stage, since the monkeys do respond differentially to the living cage environment and the test environment. This difference persists essentially without change into later phases. By the second month of life the differentiation of the surrogates has proceeded to a point where the level of distress vocalizations is reliably lower with the familiar surrogate than with the test object when both are available for contact. The monkeys continue to cling readily to both devices, however, and derive substantial emotional reassurance from either. At this age they are also reassured by both

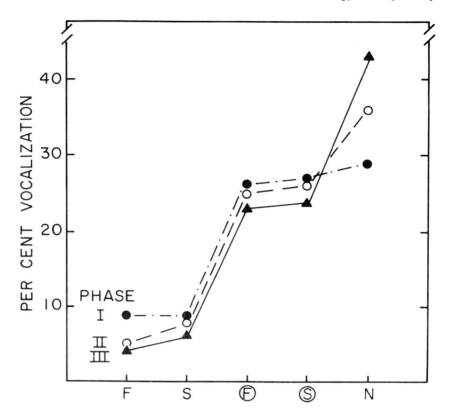

FIGURE 6   Percentage of total distress vocalizations in each object condition for the combined environments

surrogates in non-claspable form, as compared to the empty test chambers. The familiar surrogate is a more effective source of reassurance than the stranger when both are shielded in plastic, at least as measured by heart rate. The third month brings an even larger separation between the empty test chamber and all other conditions. There is a suggestion that 'emptiness' has become an aversive condition, even when the empty environment is a familiar one, although the empty familiar environment continues to be more effective than the empty test environment. The familiar surrogate shows a slight increase in effectiveness relative to the stranger when both are available for contact, but when they are encased in plastic the difference is about the same in the third month of testing as in the first month.

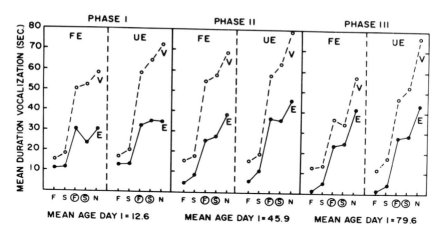

FIGURE 7 Mean duration of distress vocalizations in familiar (*FE*) and unfamiliar (*UE*) environments by monkeys raised in enclosed cages (*E*) or in cages with clear plastic fronts (*V*)

Let us turn now to the effect of rearing conditions. Our concern in establishing the visual and enclosed rearing groups was to collect some preliminary information on how the general perceptual context in which the infant/mother relationship was embedded influenced the strength and specificity of attachment. Although data are currently available for only eight of the ten animals planned for the visual group, the results suggest a substantial difference between groups. The findings on duration of vocalization are shown for the first three phases in Figure 7. The pattern of effects is similar in the two groups, but the results suggest an earlier and sharper differentiation of test conditions by the animals reared in the more complex and variable visual environment. In general, the largest intergroup differences occur in the unfamiliar environment when it contains no objects.

JAY S. ROSENBLATT

5 Some Features of Early Behavioural Development in Kittens[*]

We have been engaged in the study of some features of the early development of behaviour in newly born kittens. The object of these studies was to examine the earliest appearance of various adaptive behaviour patterns and to trace their development during the litter period. These studies were initiated in the early 1950s. At that time many investigators believed, following the writings of Scott (1958, 1962) and studies by Fuller, Easler, and Banks (1950) and James and Cannon (1952), that (a) early advances in behaviour were based largely upon the maturation of reflexes and sensory-motor abilities, and (b) that learning entered into behavioural development some-what later – e.g., in the third week in the dog and after proportionate delays in other small mammals. This is known as the 'critical period' theory. We differed from Scott: our view, with respect to the social development of kittens, was expressed as follows (Schneirla and Rosenblatt, 1963):

In the social development of the cat, we are led to the idea that striking changes in the essential progression are grounded not only in the growth-dependent processes of maturation but also, at the same time, in oppor-tunities for experience and learning arising in the standard female-litter situation. This conception of social ontogeny encourages stressing not just one or a few chronologically marked changes in behaviour patterns, but rather indicates that normally each age period is crucial for the development of particular aspects in a complex progressive pattern of adjustment.

Our initial study on kittens was an examination of the contribution of experience during various phases of suckling and related social development.

* The research reported in this article was supported by grants from the National Science Foundation and the Rockefeller Foundation to Dr T.C. Schnierla, and from the United States Public Health Service (MH-16744, MH-08604) to Dr J.S. Rosenblatt. The latter wishes to acknowledge Dr Gerald Turkewitz' contribution to the research and to thank Mr Robert J. Woll for allowing him to use the results of his study

Kittens were isolated from the mother and littermates for periods ranging from one week to forty-five days, at various times during the two-month suckling period, and reared with a brooder and artificial nipple that provided milk when suckled. To test the effects of the period of isolation upon suckling and other social behaviour, the isolates were returned to their litters and observed for several days until their behaviour had become stable. The results of this study, presented in several reports (Rosenblatt, Turkewitz, and Schneirla, 1961; Schneirla and Rosenblatt, 1961), indicated that every period was important for the normal development of suckling and social behaviour. Upon their return to their litters after a period in isolation, kittens showed the effects of their isolation in being unable to adjust to the changes in suckling and general social behaviour that had occurred in the litter during their absence. After short periods of isolation, particularly those which occurred early, kittens eventually adapted to the new situation in the litter. However, with prolonged separation, particularly during periods when advances among the littermates were based upon the development of more complex suckling and social relationships between the kittens and the mother and among the kittens themselves, the task of adapting to the mother and littermates became too difficult for the isolates, who lacked the experience for the adjustment. These results argued against any particular period as being critical for the development of social behaviour, as exemplified in the suckling pattern of the kitten. Our findings suggested that learning enters into behavioural development early in ontogeny, a view that has been borne out by many studies on a variety of mammals during the past ten years (Rosenblatt, 1971). Moreover, what kittens learn at each stage is related to those activities which are functionally significant and is based upon the maturational status of their sensory systems, motor abilities, motivational processes, and integrative capacities. Learning cannot, therefore, be arbitrarily imposed upon kittens without consideration of these factors.

With this view in mind we undertook to study two patterns of behaviour, which appear early in the behavioural ontogeny of kittens and are functionally significant from the beginning.

SUCKLING AND HOME ORIENTATION IN KITTENS

Studies on the development of suckling and home orientation in newly born kittens will be described briefly in the remainder of this paper; these studies have been reported more fully elsewhere (Schneirla, Rosenblatt, and Tobach, 1963; Rosenblatt, Turkewitz, and Schneirla, 1969). Before describing our studies, however, it is necessary to describe the setting in which these behaviour patterns develop in order to indicate their functional significance in

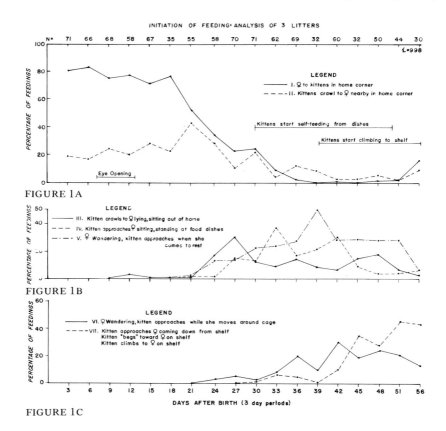

FIGURE 1A

FIGURE 1B

FIGURE 1C

the litter situation and their relationship to the general maturational status of
the kitten at various ages.

*(a) General Survey of Behavioural Interactions in the Litter during the First
Two Months, with Special Reference to Suckling*

In the laboratory, mothers and their litters exhibit a regular sequence of
behavioural changes during the first two months, several aspects of which are
depicted in the series of graphs in Figure 1. The graphs are aligned to permit
comparisons of changes during each of the age periods. For our present
purpose the end of the third week marks the beginning of an important series
of changes with which we shall be concerned. At this time the early mode of
feeding begins to decline (Figure 1A), and a new series of feeding relationships develops in rapid succession (Figures 1B and 1C). Nursing, which has

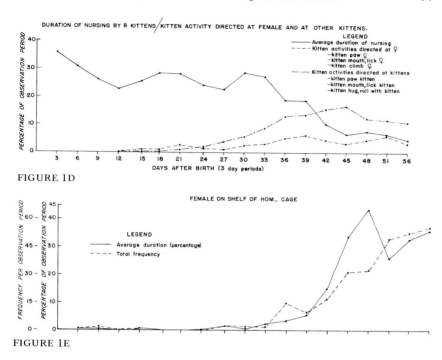

FIGURE 1D

FIGURE 1E

FIGURE 1   Summary of observations of feeding and other behaviours in three litters of kittens over the first two months. *A, B,* and *C* show the mode of initiating feeding at various phases, *D* shows nursing and play activity among the kittens and by kittens directed at the mother, and *E* shows shelf-mounting behaviour by the mother

been confined largely to the home region, begins to occur more and more frequently throughout the cage. At the same time the initiative in feeding gradually shifts from the mother to the kittens: in the early period feedings are initiated by the mother approaching the kittens, arousing them by licking, adopting the nursing position, and allowing the kitten to grasp the nipples and suckle. After the third week, the kittens leave the home region, approach the female at a distance, nuzzle, grasp nipples, and suckle. Closely associated with this change is the appearance and rapid increase of play activity among the kittens and by the kittens directed at the mother (Figure 1D).

The relatively simple social relationship, including the feeding relationship, between the mother and the kittens during the first three weeks rapidly changes after the third week, into a complex one involving greater variety and complexity of activities and subtlety of perception in the social interaction during feeding and other behaviour. Social interactions among the kittens themselves show a similar pattern of development. In addition, the kittens' relation to their non-social environment, that is the living cage in this study, also undergoes development that is inseparable from the development of social behaviour. Confinement to the limited space of the home region, in which all of their activities were carried out during the first three weeks, gives way as kittens move freely about the entire cage, their movements being determined less by the cage region and more by the social activity in which they are engaged.

It would be interesting to pursue the implications of these changes in kitten behaviour for the mother-young relationship. Our observations indicate that in response to the play activity of the kittens the mother begins to leave the litter (for a shelf located 18 inches above the cage floor) for long periods and at frequent intervals (Figure 1 E). When she leaves the kittens alone for these long periods, the kittens turn to other sources of food that are available in the cage and suckling from the mother begins to decline (Figure 1 D) as they begin to wean themselves from her. Further discussion of these developments, however, would lead us away from the discussion of suckling and home orientation.

Suckling and home orientation represent the principal adaptations of the newly born kitten to the main features of its early environment, namely, the mother and the surrounding environment of the home site. An analysis of these early patterns of behaviour reveals the behavioural capacities of the developing kitten.

(b) Suckling

Suckling is initiated shortly after parturition in the 'post-partum resting interval' which we have described (Schneirla, Rosenblatt, and Tobach, 1963), as is typical in many mothers. A significant development takes place, however, on the second or third day, when suckling has been established and occurs at regular intervals, several times every two hours. At each feeding individual kittens can be seen headed for particular nipple regions; each kitten establishes a preference for a specific set of nipples, the upper and lower ones at either the posterior, middle, or anterior positions on the mammary surface of the mother as she lies on her side. The nipple position preferences of a litter of four kittens is shown in Table I. Kittens, A, B, and C showed an early development of preferences for nipple positions II, III, and IV in that order, while kitten D showed nearly equal preference for nipple positions II and III. By the end of the second day more than fifty per cent of a group of twenty-seven kittens have established nipple position preferences and by the end of the third day the percentage has risen to eighty-five.

TABLE I The frequencies of suckling at the different nipple positions by four kittens of a litter during the first 12 days. The nipple positions are numbered I to IV, anterior to posterior

Day	Kitten A/nipple pair				Kitten B/nipple pair				Kitten C/nipple pair				Kitten D/nipple pair			
	I	II	III	IV	I	II	III	IV	I	II	III	IV	I	II	III	IV
1	4	3	2	3	0	7	1	4	0	2	2	9	1	2	6	1
2	1	7	4				11	5			1	14	1	7	4	
3		35	5			1	11				1	17		10	2	
4		17	2				18	1			3	16		7	4	
5		21	2	1		1	27				3	25		3	14	
6		8	3				17				1	16		6	5	
7		7	3	1			7				1	6		4	6	
8		9	4				13	1		2	4	21		10	2	
9		9	7	2		3	18	1		3	9	14		14	12	2
10		3	3			1	8	2		1	2	10		5		
11		12	12	6		1	12	2		4	6	14		7	13	2
12		9	7	2		6	8	6		1	6	11		9	10	
Totals	5	140	54	15	0	20	152	31	0	13	39	173	2	84	68	5

With respect to suckling, therefore, learning enters very early into be-havioural development as recent studies on puppies (Stanley, Bacon, and Fehr, 1970), rat young (Thoman, Wetzel, and Levine, 1968), and monkey and human infants (Lipsitt, 1967; Mason and Harlow, 1958) have also shown. We have attempted to produce nipple position preferences experimentally in newly born kittens that were removed from their mothers at birth and placed in isolation (Woll and Rosenblatt, unpublished). The kittens were presented with a brooder, which was essentially a flat bunting-covered surface, at a forty-five degree angle from the floor, from which two nipples protruded spaced two inches apart at their bases much as the nipples are on the mother. To study the possible stimulus basis for learning to distinguish one nipple from another and to suckle differentially from the two nipples, the nipple bases of our experimental feeder were given two different textures (i.e., raised dot vs. concentric circles), or two different odours. Kittens learned very rapidly to distinguish between the two 'nipple positions' on the basis of either the tactile or olfactory differences and they preferred the nipple position from which they received milk over the one which had a blind nipple. Their learning and preference could be measured by the amount of time they spent nuzzling at the base of each of the two nipples (Figure 2): olfactory dis-crimination was clearly established by the third day and tactile discrimination even earlier, on the second day. Kittens were placed on the milk-filled nipple after they had indicated their preference, but by the fourth day (and even earlier, on the second and third days in most kittens) they were able to grasp the nipple in their mouths by themselves.

In addition to providing evidence of early learning in kittens in relation to a functionally significant activity, the establishment of these preferences, based, presumably, upon subtle differences among the nipples in tactile, olfactory, and perhaps thermal stimuli, indicates an important turning point in the kittens' development. The kittens' initial suckling is based upon their responses to low intensity tactile, olfactory, and perhaps thermal stimuli which guide them indiscriminately to any one or several of the nipple posi-tions, and to the nipples themselves which elicit mouth grasping and sucking. The speed with which the kittens initiate suckling after birth testifies to the effectiveness of their initial nipple localization and mouth grasping responses and to the channelling effect of the mother's mammary surface. But the establishment of nipple position preferences indicates that many of the stimuli which previously were effective in leading the kittens to the nipples and in eliciting nipple grasping, have become ineffective. Kittens often pass by several non-preferred nipples on their way to their own preferred nipples just as they give up nuzzling at the base of the blind nipple in our brooder and turn to the base of the milk-filled nipple. The stimuli to which the kittens

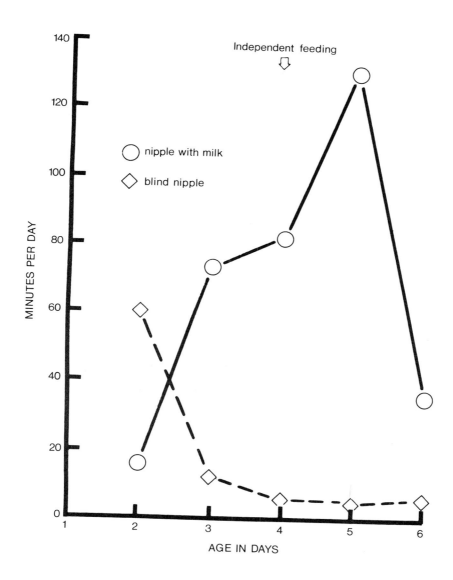

FIGURE 2 The amount of time a brooder-reared kitten spent nuzzling at nipple bases differing in olfactory stimulation. One nipple base was associated with a nipple that provided milk and the other was associated with a blind nipple

respond in locating their preferred nipples may not be different from those to which they responded earlier (determined by their dependence upon the non-visual sensory systems since the kittens' eyes are sealed for the first week or so of life). Moreover, whether or not these earlier stimuli elicit approach or withdrawal reactions is an important factor in how rapidly they are incorporated into the newly developing nipple localization pattern. But the features of these stimuli to which the kittens now respond are different. What these features are and how they differ among the nipples cannot yet be stated, but it is quite clear that each kitten's use of distinguishing features of the nipples is based upon its individual experience during the first days of suckling.

With more or less clearly discriminated nipple preferences established, kittens begin to develop routes to the nipples; in the brooder these routes are clearly observable and on the mother's body certain landmarks along the route to the nipples can be noted, as for example, the mother's outstretched fore- and hindlegs, which, followed closely in the direction towards her body, lead kittens to particular nipple positions. During the first three weeks, therefore, when gross observation of nursing reveals no apparent progress in suckling, closer observation indicates that kittens are establishing and extending their routes to their preferred nipples. The starting phase of the path to the nipple, even in their early period, occurs, occasionally, when the kitten is out of contact with the mother but nearby in the home region Figure 1 A).

Many features of this and subsequent developments in suckling can be seen in relation to the brooder and have been observed in kittens that suckled regularly and exclusively from mothers that were immobilized by anaesthesia (Koepke and Pribram, 1971).

The onset of visually guided behaviour, a gradual process extending from the fourteenth day to late in the fourth week, introduces a major change in the suckling pattern by enabling kittens to perceive the mother at a distance. Increasingly after the third week, the starting phase of the suckling pattern follows after the kittens have engaged in prolonged visual following of the mother as she moves about the cage. When she comes to rest, the kittens initiate their suckling approaches to her and, when close to her, they resort to non-visual stimuli for locating the nipple. The succession of increasingly complex modes of initiating suckling by kittens, shown in Figure 1 (c and d), indicates the further progress which is made during this period. With vision now an avenue for perceiving the mother, many aspects of her behaviour, which previously could not be important to the kittens now become so, and suckling is increasingly dependent upon a broader and more complex social interaction between the kitten and the mother.

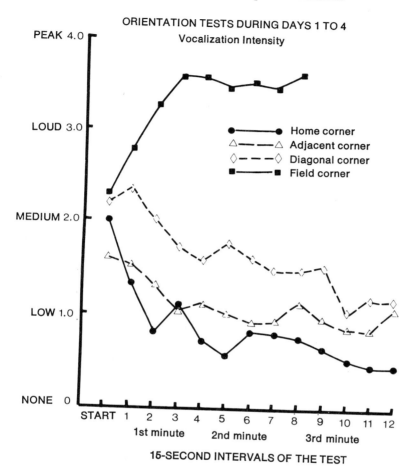

FIGURE 3A The intensity of vocalization during three-minute tests in the cage corners and two-minute tests in the field at various age periods

(c) Home Orientation

Confinement to the home site during the first three weeks, an important feature of suckling, as we have seen, is not based simply or perhaps at all upon the inability of kittens to locomote sufficiently to leave this region. It is based upon the development of an 'attachment' by kittens to features of the home. Evidence for this attachment can be found in two kinds of behaviour

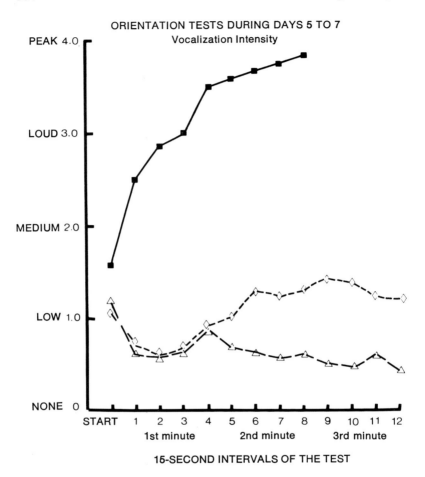

FIGURE 3B The curve for the home corner during the period from the 5th to the 7th day has been omitted

which kittens exhibit, which together we have called 'home orientation.' The first of these and the one which appears earlier in development, starting around the first to fourth day, is the vocalization which kittens produce when they are replaced in the home region after they have been removed and provoked to cry. Such vocalizations can be rated with respect to their intensity on a scale from one to four, with the low and high values representing low- and high-intensity vocalization respectively. In three-minute tests

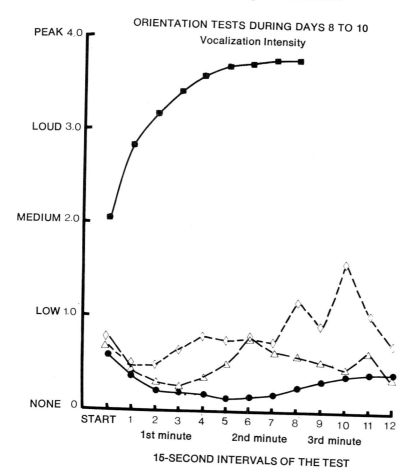

FIGURE 3C   Days eight to ten

replacing kittens in the home region, and in the region of the adjacent corner
and the corner diagonally opposite from the home region (diagonal corner)
vocalizations differ, being lowest in the home and highest in the more distant
diagonal corner (Figure 3). Higher intensities of vocalization are indicative of
disturbance and in a region completely different from the home cage where
kittens are most disturbed — such as a freshly washed field — their vocalizations are the most intense. After the fourth day (i.e., fifth to seventh

day, and eighth to tenth day), kittens continue to vocalize at low in-tensities in the home but they continue to vocalize at a somewhat greater intensity in the adjacent corner and at a still greater intensity in the diagonal corner; the most intense vocalizations occur in the field. In fact, after the fourth day kittens vocalize in the home only for a brief time at the moment they are replaced. Within a short time they become quiet and often fall asleep. The home region is therefore a place in which they are comforted, while regions outside the home produce disturbance. This probably is the reason why kittens never leave the home region on their own accord for nearly the first three weeks after birth.

The other behaviour which kittens exhibit in relation to the home region is illustrated in Figures 4 and 5. At five days of age, when placed in the adjacent corner of the cage, kittens begin to crawl in the direction of the home region and within a short time (i.e., one to two minutes) they enter the home and soon fall asleep. When they are placed in the home region at this age, they crawl a bit, then come to rest and fall asleep. Finding their way to the home region from the diagonal corner is a more difficult task for kittens and it appears later in development than pathtaking to the home from the adjacent corner. Nevertheless by the fourteenth day, as depicted in Figure 5 which shows the orientation to the home from the diagonal corner of a twenty-day-old kitten, kittens begin to find their way to the home when they are initially placed in the diagonal corner.

We have done experiments which indicate that the olfactory characteristics of the home region, most likely parturitive fluids initially and deposits from the fur and body of the mother and kittens later, distinguish this region from other regions of the home cage and from the field situation (Rosenblatt, Turkewitz, and Schneirla, 1969). We have proposed that these deposits are distributed on the floor of the cage in a gradient, spread by the mother chiefly, and that the high point of the gradient is in the home region. Our studies suggest that kittens follow sections of the gradient from the adjacent and diagonal corners to reach the home but, in the home, movement outward in any direction leads the kitten into regions that contain less of the olfactory stimuli. Since this produces a disturbance in the kittens it is unlikely that they will continue to move away from the home but instead, having begun, they will turn back into the home; this, in fact, is what occurs.

Around the fourteenth day, however, at the beginning of visual function-ing, the use of olfactory stimuli to find the home is supplemented by the use of visual cues. Initially this development, which as we have seen plays an important role in the development of more complex forms of suckling, also leads to an improvement in orientation to the home. Instead of following the

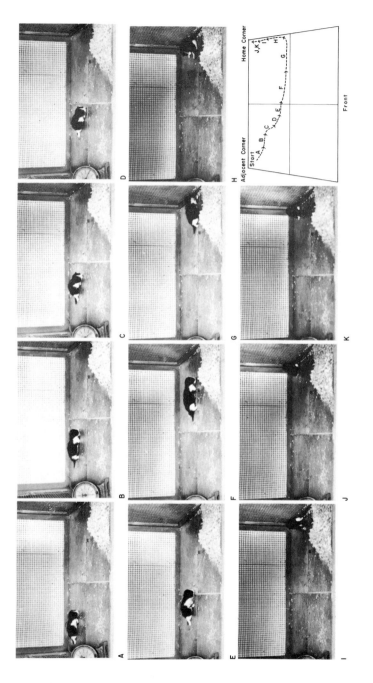

FIGURE 4   Home orientation of a 5-day-old kitten placed in the adjacent corner of the home cage. The home region is at the right and the path taken by the kitten is shown in the drawn figure

earlier roundabout path to the home dictated by the distribution of olfactory deposits on the floor of the cage, kittens walk directly towards the home.

But, since home orientation is dependent upon a comforting effect of the home on kittens, and since this in turn appears to be a function of the home's special olfactory characteristics, then as kittens gain comfort from visually perceived features of the litter situation, as, for example, the mother and littermates, or even from the sight of the home cage, the importance of olfactory stimuli in the home diminishes. This begins to occur around the eighteenth day, starting first when kittens are placed in the home and later when they are placed in the other cage corners. They begin to leave the home region when placed there, return to it again, then leave, vacillating in their behaviour at first. We have already seen that when the mother is present the kittens approach her and often suckle, thus the behaviour of leaving the home region seen in orientation tests is normally reinforced by the visually-based attraction to the mother when she is present. The home-oriented behaviour of kittens gradually wanes, and they freely leave the home and wander around the cage, gaining their comfort from interacting with the mother and litter-mates (Rheingold and Eckerman, 1971). There is some indication that the new visually-based spatial orientation of kittens gives rise to special centres of orientation but these are related to specific functions: for example, kittens tend to use special cage regions for sleeping, others for elimination functions, etc.

Thus, while the onset of visual functioning is the basis for the broadening of the kittens' suckling pattern and an increase in its complexity, the effect on the early pattern of spatial orientation (i.e., home orientation) is to lead to its disappearance. Of course, in a larger sense, the decline of the restriction upon their movements which olfactory-based home orientation imposes upon the kittens ultimately enables them also to broaden the range and complexity of spatial orientation.

GENERAL RELEVANCE OF THESE STUDIES

These studies stand as evidence of the early appearance of learning in the behavioural development of kittens and of its close relationship to the kitten's maturational status, at each stage. The successful discovery of early learning in these studies stands in contrast to previous failures to demonstrate learning in newborn puppies, failures which have now been turned into successes by methods similar to those we employed. The principal factor which has enabled us, as well as others, to find evidence of early learning was the selection for study of functionally relevant behaviour patterns in the

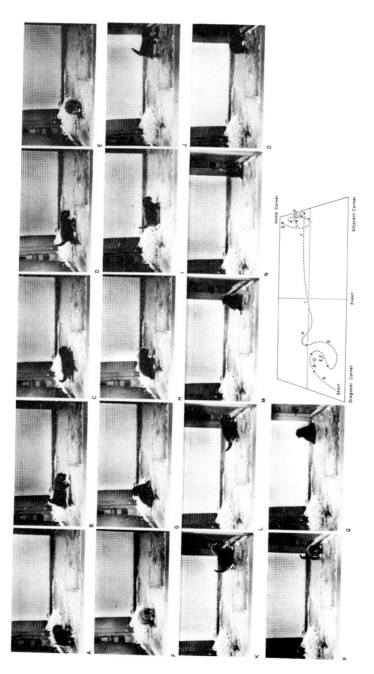

FIGURE 5 Home orientation from the diagonal corner of the home cage by a 20-day-old kitten. The drawn figure shows the path taken from the diagonal corner to the home

newborn. In the kitten these are represented by suckling and home orientation; in other species the relevant behaviour patterns may be different.

The data themselves are of some interest in another context. The kitten is representative of many other species with altricial young, in which the mother builds a nest or establishes a home site for delivery and care of her young. There is growing evidence in many of these species that the newborn form a pattern of orientation to the nest site in addition to the formation of a suckling pattern in relation to the mother. Thus the typical conditions of their early life give rise to a division of attachment between the mother and the home site among kittens and other newborn altricial mammals. By contrast, among most subhuman primates the mother functions as both the 'nest site' and the suckling object as a consequence of the fact that she carries the infant around with her on her body at all times. This circumstance must certainly lead to different types of development in the infant monkey, for example, and the newly born kitten. Functions which are initially separate in the kitten, only gradually converging upon the mother comfort-source as the suckling object and visual orientation, are for the infant monkey formed in relation to the same object right from the beginning.

Even as adults, cats and monkeys differ in the degree to which they are dependent upon proximity to species mates, the cat being much less so than the monkey. In order to explore the usefulness of animal studies for an understanding of human behaviour we must be prepared to incorporate contrasting patterns of behavioural development, found in different mammals as well as seemingly similar ones, into our theoretical framework.

SOCIAL ORGANIZATION

IRVEN DEVORE, MELVIN J. KONNER

6 Infancy in Hunter-Gatherer Life: An Ethological Perspective*

Since this paper is the only report on studies of a 'free-ranging *human* primate,' it may seem somewhat curious in the context of this volume. Nor can the studies reported here be called 'ethological' in the same sense as those undertaken by, for example, Eibl-Eibesfeldt (1970). Yet our studies have been strongly influenced by the concerns and theoretical issues raised by ethological studies, and the definition of the field 'ethology' becomes less precise every year (Lockhard, 1971). Richard Borshay Lee and DeVore began the 'San (Bushman) Project'[1] in 1963, not only with prior experience in non-human primate studies, but also with a determination to gather data on hunter-gatherers as objectively and quantitatively as possible. For example, in the first period of the study the observers neither accepted food and water from, nor offered it to, San (!Kung) groups residing nearby. While this did not ingratiate us to the local San, it enabled us to gather quantitative data on food consumption, residence patterns, group movement, and so forth in a way that would not have been possible had we engaged in the more common

* The original field study (1963-4) was financed by a grant from the US National Science Foundation. Since 1967 it has been financed primarily by grants from the US National Institutes of Mental Health (MH 13611), with additional support from the Wenner-Gren Foundation for Anthropological Research and the Milton Fund (Harvard). We would like to acknowledge gratefully the support of these foundations, as well as the support and collaboration of the following institutions: Harvard University, University of Capetown Medical School, the South African Institute for Medical Research, and the Council for Scientific and Industrial Research of South Africa.

    Only one of us (DeVore) attended the conference at McMaster. Following the conference Melvin Konner had returned from 20 months of research on infancy among the Bushmen, a topic that seemed particularly pertinent to the concerns of the conference. The second portion of the paper is a partial description of Konner's data.

    The authors wish to express their thanks to Dr T. Berry Brazelton, Professor Jerome Kagan, Dr N.G. Blurton-Jones, Professor John Whiting, Nancy DeVore, and especially to Charles Super, and Sara Harkness. Their comments on an earlier draft of this paper, especially the portions on infancy, resulted in many improvements in the final version. The authors, however, are solely responsible for the views expressed

1 Although these people are traditionally referred to as 'Bushmen,' scholars have recently replaced this term with the non-pejorative 'San.'

pattern of convivial communality that has characterized most field work among hunter-gatherer peoples. Further, the technique of non-interfering observation was practical at a time when none of us had learned the language. Finally, these studies of the San are ethological in spirit in their emphasis on the description of observed behaviour patterns, rather than reliance on the more common anthropological technique of the interview.

As the project has progressed, eight of the field workers have become fluent in the local language, and we have used the interview extensively. But we continue to emphasize the collection of data uncontaminated either by the fallibility of recollection, or by the tendency of the informants to shape their answers to the expected response· of the interviewer or by the strictures of their own value system. (It is both curious and sad that much of the popular 'ethological literature' becomes anecdotal and inferential when it turns to considerations of human behaviour and institutions.) This is not to imply that interview data are not valuable; obviously men perceive the world through cognitive filters, and structure their lives by the manipulation of symbols. But this kind of information alone, abundant in the monographs of social anthropology, is at best one-sided, and may be very misleading with respect to the kinds of information an ecologist or ethologist would value. To take an example: the !Kung group of San in the Kalahari are preoccupied with food — its acquisition, distribution, and consumption. Their traditional greeting is often followed by the declaration 'father (or mother), I'm starving!' Yet our data indicate that these same persons are among the best fed in the world. That they have food *anxieties* is perhaps significant in understanding the attitude of hunter-gatherers toward an unpredictable subsistence base, but to conclude from this attitude that they are chronically *malnourished* (as has often been done in hunter-gatherer studies) is unwarranted (e.g., Lee, 1968; Sahlins, 1968).

THE HUNTER-GATHERER PAST

It is reasonable to ask why a small, remote population of hunter-gatherers on the edge of the Kalahari Desert of Africa should be singled out for intensive study, and why we feel that this population may have more theoretical interest for understanding the basis of human behaviour, development, and society than other populations. The answer, of course, is that all mankind lived a hunter-gatherer existence for more than 99 per cent of the some three million years cultural man has occupied this planet. Even if we ignore our more remote hominid ancestors, we see that *Homo sapiens* assumed a modern form at least fifty thousand years before the species began to domesticate plants and animals or modify the environment in any significant way.

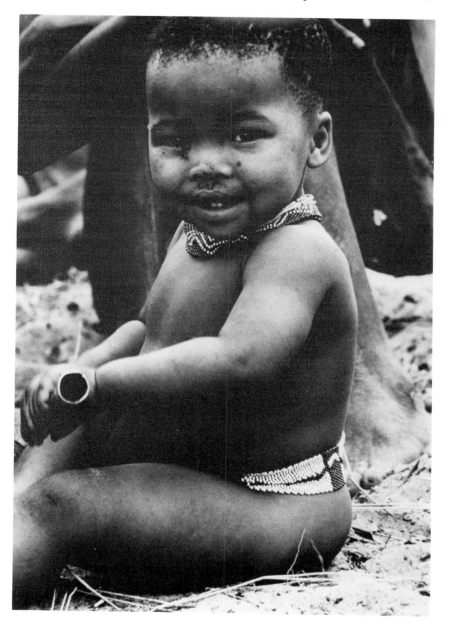

FIGURE 1   A !Kung baby at play (photo: Irven DeVore)

In terms of time, the human line has been separated from its nearest primate ancestors by at least five million years, quite possibly much longer, and throughout this period we adapted and evolved as hunter-gatherers. The 'agricultural revolution' began about ten thousand years ago, and by the time of Christ, eight thousand years later, agriculturists and pastoralists had replaced hunter-gatherers over only about one-half of the globe. Today what was once the universal method of human subsistence is confined to isolated remnants of peoples in refuge habitats. But the last few thousand years are but a moment in evolutionary time, and it seems worthwhile to ask whether the hunter-gatherer way of life, that was so instrumental in shaping our bodies, may not have left its imprint on our psyches as well – a suggestion elaborated by the psychiatrist D.A. Hamburg (1963). Human patterns of aggression, of affection, of reaction to stress, and the structure of family and group life, were all fashioned in a hunting and gathering context, and in our studies we are seeking to understand this way of life as completely as possible.

There are obvious problems in this approach. Although it was a conceit of nineteenth century anthropology to seek living relics of our own past among the 'primitive peoples' of the world, arranging them along a scale of development from the benighted aborigine to the exalted Victorian Englishman, one need hardly argue today the futility of such an attempt. Yet one can still encounter (in a recent medical journal) such statements as 'of course the Bushmen have only a rudimentary language containing about fifty words.' Suffice it to say that the San of the Kalahari Desert are fully modern, psychologically and physically, and their behaviour and institutions have continued to evolve in parallel to those of people around them. One finds among them the full range of human emotional and intellectual potential. Our interest in this people, then, is not that of the entomologist who discovers an extinct insect perfectly preserved in amber, but an interest in the degree to which they represent universally human behavioural and social responses to the hunter-gatherer way of life. By this criterion we are just as interested in the adaptation and behaviour of all hunter-gatherer peoples, but the Kalahari San do represent the largest intact population available for study.

In a paper as brief as this very little attention can be given to the problem of comparison between different hunter-gatherer societies, but many of the modern studies are compared in *Man the Hunter* (Lee and DeVore, 1968). This volume was the result of an international conference of some seventy-five scholars who met to reassess current studies of hunter-gatherers throughout the world, and explore the implications of these studies for social anthropology, human biology, archaeology, demography, and ecology. How generally representative of hunter-gatherers the San in our studies have been can best be appreciated by reference to that volume. Not unexpectedly, the more environmental variables are held constant, the more comparable the social institutions of hunter-gatherers. Tropical Old World hunger-gatherers seem very similar in certain basic ways, and some of these are indicated below. More specialized hunter-gatherers such as arctic hunters, a recent and divergent adaptation, show important contrasts, (but even they are similar in many important respects). Since human evolution took place in the Old World tropics, under climatic conditions and in association with plants and animals quite comparable to what they are at present, generalizations based on hunter-gatherers in this region have the advantage of introducing the smallest number of extraneous variables.

One problem when using contemporary hunter-gatherers for prehistoric reconstruction cannot be easily overcome: contemporary hunter-gatherers live in refuge habitats. Since the beginning of the neolithic, agriculturalists have been steadily expanding at the expense of the hunters; today hunter-gatherers are found in areas either very remote, or unattractive to agriculturalists and pastoralists. The more favourable habitats have long since been appropriated by populations with larger, more cohesive, more aggressive social systems. Jungles, deserts, and tundras often pose difficult problems of survival, leading observers to assume that the lives of contemporary hunter-gatherers (and therefore the lives of our own ancestors) were a constant struggle for survival — lives that were, in Hobbes' words, 'nasty, brutish, and short.' These conclusions, and their implications, are very much mistaken, as indicated below.

THE SAN PROJECT

Our studies have been centered on a population of about 1600 !Kung San living in western Ngamiland, Botswana, near the border of Namibia (South West Africa). Although only a small fraction still live entirely by hunting and gathering, there are about 55,000 persons who can be considered (linguistically) 'San' living in Botswana, Namibia, and Angola (Lee, 1965). About 13,000 of these are traditionally called the !Kung, although in the area of our studies (!angwa) they refer to themselves as the 'Zun/wasi.' (The ! and / symbols denote palatal and dental clicks respectively, two of four such clicks in the language. The clicks are a linguistic feature that set apart the South African 'click languages' from other language families.)

Lee and DeVore began the study in 1963-64, Lee spending seventeen and DeVore four months in the field. We returned in 1967 with a larger group of anthropologists in such fields as medicine, nutrition, and demography, to undertake a wide-ranging series of investigations that are still in progress.

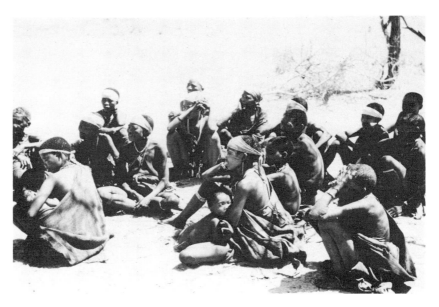

FIGURE 2   Part of a San band in repose (photo: Irven DeVore)

These include studies of hunting and gathering techniques, archaeology, demography, migration and population genetics, nutrition and general health, infant growth and development, child-rearing practices, settlement patterns, and the ritual curing trance. For long-term demographic studies, the sample of persons for whom we have basic biographical information now numbers 850 (although only about 600 persons are resident in the study areas at any time); blood samples and birth and marital data have been collected from a total of 2000 individuals. The publications by some 25 research workers since 1963 are too numerous to mention here (a bibliography will be supplied on request), nor can this brief description indicate more than a few selected aspects of !Kung life.

The !angwa region, where we have centred our studies, still contains a viable hunter-gatherer population because the climate and soils of the area are poorly suited for cultivation. Situated on the northwestern fringe of the Kalahari desert, and surrounded by a waterless zone, the !angwa region was buffered from incursions by either Bantu or European pastoralists and agriculturists until a small group of Herero cattle herders settled there in 1925. Today the !Kung share all but the smallest of their eight permanent waterholes with about 350 Hereros (together with several thousand head of

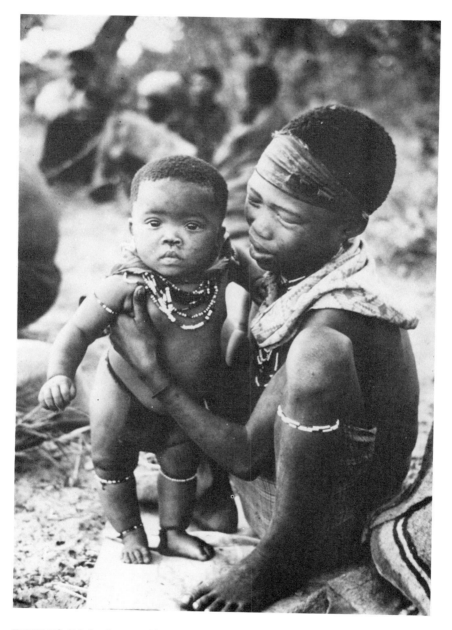

FIGURE 3 It is hard to pose if you cannot stand (photo: Irven DeVore)

livestock), and assimilation of the !Kung as satellites of Herero cattle posts is accelerating rapidly.

It is traditional in anthropology to view hunter-gatherers as living in tightly knit male-oriented bands, where kinship is traced through the male line (patri-lineality) and residence is with the husband's kin (patrilocality) (e.g., Radcliffe-Brown, 1931; Service, 1966). The band was thought to be highly territorial, and very protective of hunting areas, water sources, and so on. While such patri-lineal, patrilocal, territorial bands may have existed among some hunter-gatherer peoples, this characterization stems in no small part from armchair theorizing: as the primary food providers, the men would have to dominate hunter-gatherer life; they would co-operate in hunting, drive other hunters away, and lead the band to areas where game was plentiful. Further, it seemed apparent to even trained observers that hunter-gatherer life must be harsh — their nomadic travels and lack of material goods seemed evidence enough that the hunters (and, by implication, our own ancestors) lived in grinding poverty. Such conceptualizations could scarcely be further from conditions we found among the !Kung groups. There are no organized 'bands,' but clusters of families at campsites whose composition changes almost daily; nuclear and extended families move freely over an area of a hundred square miles or more, camping with relatives and kinsmen throughout the region (e.g., Lee, 1972). Kinship is traced equally through the husband's and wife's families, and residence, like all aspects of group structure, is fluid and subject to frequent changes. Far from defending territories, in this free-flowing popula-tion the very concept is meaningless. While there are allegedly 'owners' of certain waterholes, their claim to ownership is often recent, disputed, and, in any case, not enforced. Finally, far from living at a substandard nutritional level, the San are able to maintain themselves well above minimum standard nutritional levels, even in drought years, with a modest work week of only two or three days per adult, with older persons, children, and adolescents rarely participating significantly in the food quest (e.g., Lee, 1969).

Earlier students of hunter-gatherer life were not prepared to gather quanti-tative data on work levels and caloric intake, and they significantly under-estimated the role of women in the food quest. Modern investigators have often remarked that peoples such as the pygmies of the Ituri forest, the Australian aborigines, and the San (!Kung) might better be called 'gatherer-hunters,' and indeed we have found that women contribute from 50 to 80 per cent of foodstuffs by weight, depending on the group, the time of year, etc. More important, while vegetable foods can be gathered regularly and

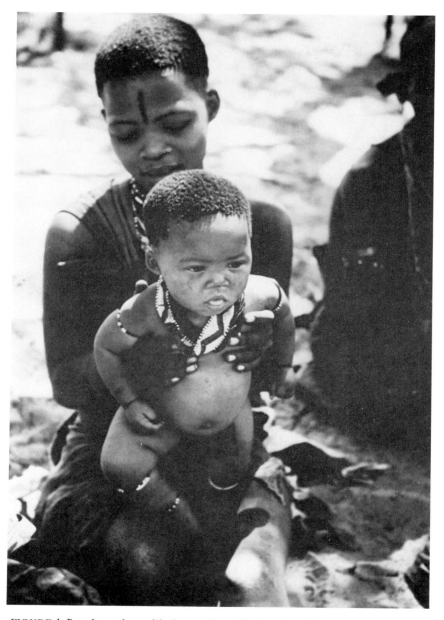

FIGURE 4 Proud mother with her well-nourished and well-beaded infant (photo: Irven DeVore)

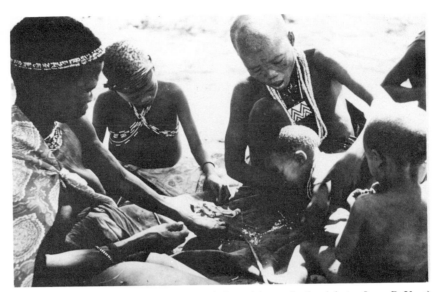

FIGURE 5 Sharing plays a predominant role in social organization (photo: Irven DeVore)

infallibly, hunting success is far from predictable; a hunter may return with a hare, an eland, or (more likely) no meat at all. We find no reason to suppose that the relative contribution to the economy by women was ever less, in the past, than it is among contemporary hunter-gatherers. Ironically, however, the only tools a woman needs to collect vegetable staples are a skin bag and a digging stick — neither of which are likely to be preserved in archaeological sites. The elaborate hunting equipment of the men, however, will always be well represented in the form of arrow heads, spear points, knives, etc. The result is an almost inescapable tendency to underestimate both vegetable foods and the economic importance of women in the interpretation of pre-historic living sites.

The staple food of the Zun/wasi of the !angwa region is in fact the remarkable mungongo nut, *Ricinodendron rautenenii* Schinz. A woman collecting mungongo nuts will bring back to camp, on the average, 12.5kg from a single day's collecting trip, and this will yield 1750g of edible nut meats. The caloric value of mungongo nuts is 600 cal/100g per edible portion (about the same as domesticated nuts such as almonds and peanuts), but mungongo nuts contain about 27 per cent protein (compared to 19 per cent in other species) (Lee, 1969).

From the above description one can characterize the Zun/wasi as a people whose work effort is modest and whose leisure time is abundant. An important key to understanding the San economy is to realize that food (and material goods) are shared, not stored. The food quest is constant, but the returns are more than adequate. Medical examinations, blood tests, and population statistics reveal the San to be well nourished and long lived. Their population density of about 0.4 persons per square mile is relatively high, compared to other estimates of hunter-gatherers living in arid regions. It is important to remember that most hunter-gatherers throughout prehistory lived in regions far *more* favoured than the Kalahari fringe – abundant in water, food plants, and game.

CHARACTERISTICS OF HUNTER-GATHERER SOCIETIES

In this brief treatment it is not possible to compare the !Kung to other tropical hunting and gathering peoples. The following characterization of the general principles of hunter-gatherer life is excerpted from a discussion of recent studies of many such groups, and the reader is directed to that discussion for evidence and details (Lee and DeVore, 1968):

First, if individuals and groups have to move around in order to get food there is an important implication: the amount of personal property has to be kept to a very low level ... a generally egalitarian system . . .

Second, the nature of the food supply keeps the living groups small, usually under fifty persons ... It is probably necessary to continually redistribute the population between bands in order to maintain food-gathering units at an effective level.

Third, the local groups as groups do not ordinarily maintain exclusive rights to resources. Variations in food supply from region to region and from year to year create a fluid situation that can best be met by flexible organizations that allow people to move from one area to another. The visiting patterns create intergroup obligations, so that the hosts in one season become the guests in another ...

Fourth, food surpluses are not a prominent feature of the small-scale society. If inventories of food on hand are minimal, then a fairly constant work effort has to be kept up throughout the year. Since everyone knows where the food is, in effect the environment itself is the storehouse; and since everyone knows the movements of everyone else, there is a lack of concern that food resources will fail or be appropriated by others.

Fifth, frequent visiting between resource areas prevents any one group from becoming too strongly attached to any single area ...

[Sixth] ... the lack of impediments in the form of personal and collective property allows a considerable degree of freedom of movement. Individuals and groups can change residence without relinquishing vital interests in land or goods, and when arguments break out it is a simple matter to part company in order to avoid serious conflict ... The resolution of conflict by fission ... may help to explain how order can be maintained in a society without superordinate means of social control.

THE CONTEXT OF INFANCY AND CHILD CARE

We were surprised to discover that, on the average, !Kung infants are spaced 4 to 5 years apart. Although !Kung women claim some knowledge of contraceptive and abortion techniques, and although infanticide is occasionally practised (e.g., in cases of congenital deformity, or when an infant is born before the previous infant can be weaned) none of these practises seem capable of explaining the long birth intervals. It is possible that prolonged, frequent, vigorous nursing suppresses ovulation more than in many populations, in which supplementary milk and/or soft foods are available for the infant. What proportion of women achieve this birth spacing, and by what means, is being investigated by Nancy Howell and Marjorie Shostak Konner. It is clear, however, that both the necessity of nursing an infant for several years, and the inability of women to carry more than one child during their food collecting rounds, serve to maintain selective pressures against more frequent birth intervals.

One result of this birth spacing, and of the small, isolated nature of San encampments, is that infants and children are rarely without adult supervision. Patricia Draper, who has studied the context of !Kung child-rearing in detail, estimates an average density in a camp of about 25 square yards per person (Draper, 1972). The central area around which the family huts are clustered is denuded of grass, bushes, or any obstruction to vision. A child in the village is within sight and hearing of all the other adults and children almost all of the time. It is into this rich social network of nurturant adults and children that the !Kung infant is born.

MATERNAL CARE IN INFANCY: AN ETHOLOGICAL PERSPECTIVE

There has been concern expressed about the recent spate of popular works on ethology, including some criticism appearing in this volume. These books purport to integrate the findings of ethology in such a way that they will be of use to professionals attempting to cope with social, pedagogical, and mental health issues, but in fact they are little more than hodge-podges of intriguing facts about animals with tacked-on, and often irresponsible, conclusions about man (e.g., Ardrey, 1961, 1966, 1970; Lorenz, 1966; Morris,

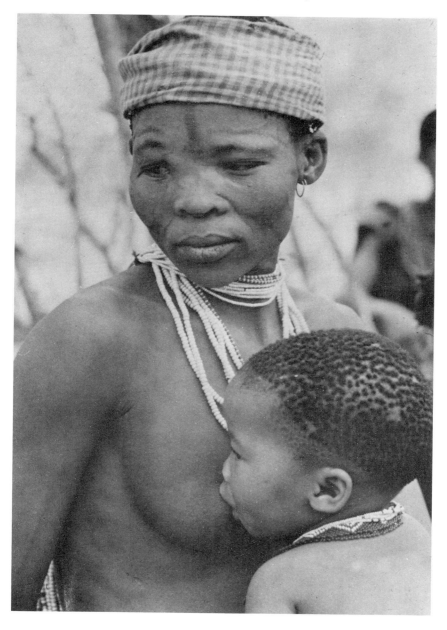

FIGURE 6 Breast feeding may continue for three to four years (photo: Irven DeVore)

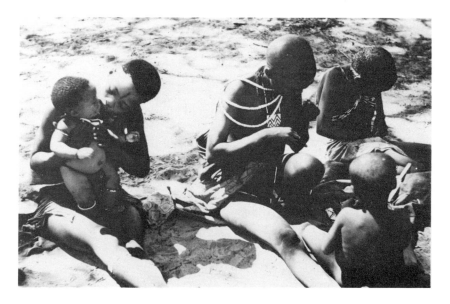

FIGURE 7 Domestic life under the Kalahari sun (photo: Irven DeVore)

1968). In this area it is gratifying to refer to at least one responsible and serious attempt to bring together a large volume of research data in a theoretical framework that is at once reasoned, elegant, and testable – the first volume of John Bowlby's *Attachment and Loss* (1969). Bowlby's volume has the added advantage of taking a clear stance in relation to the history of psychoanalytic theories of development, and, further, is derived from a body of work concerned directly with the making of child care policy.

Our work on behaviour, development, and maternal care in infancy and early childhood, though initiated before the appearance of Bowlby's monograph, is in many respects very close to its concerns, and can be seen in part as a testing ground for the validity and appropriateness of Bowlby's conceptualization.

THE BOWLBY POSITION

Briefly, Bowlby's position is as follows: the human infant, like infants of many species of birds and mammals, is born with a set of reflexive perceptuo-motor mechanisms. Though they can be blocked under experimental conditions of deprivation, given the normal, expectable environment of a newly-born member of the species, they will inevitably result in the formation of attachments to caretaking figures and subsequently, to other individuals. For Bowlby, the emphasis in the first half-year is on mechanisms involving distal receptors, such as visual-postural orientation, smiling, crying and the cessation of crying, and non-cry vocalizations. The rooting and sucking reflexes connected with feeding, and the tendency for various forms of tactile stimulation and/or suckling to be very effective in bringing about the cessation of crying and other discomfort signs, are held to be important, but not overridingly important components of the initial attachment propensity. Specifically, Bowlby is critical of 'secondary drive' theory (theory that stresses the role of satiation of hunger and the pleasure of suckling as primary reinforcers for attachment behaviour) common to many psychoanalytic conceptions, including Freud's (1920). Later in the first year, in association with the development of effective locomotion, proximity-maintaining mechanisms and attachment behaviours depending upon proximal receptors come into play. These include grasping, clinging, and scrambling and climbing on the mother, and come to include following behaviour and the use of the mother as a base for exploration.

In lieu of either learning or drive theories of the growth of love, Bowlby proposes an ethological unfolding of attachment behaviour in accord with an imperfectly understood genetic program. This behaviour system is, as it were, 'seeking' an object, in something like the way the neural mechanisms underlying imprinting in precocial birds are 'seeking,' at a certain period, a suitable object for following behaviour — with the important difference that in man and his close relatives the process is much longer (some seven months in man) and very much more gradual. (What we mean by 'seeking' is that the behaviours in question — attachment behaviours — will fully emerge, change, and function in certain predictable ways only after an appropriate object is found, and that the organism will experience considerable discomfort *until* an appropriate object is found). Because of the need for immature organisms to maintain close physical proximity to more mature members of the species, as protection against death by exposure or predation, these underlying neural mechanisms are under powerful selective pressure.

This emphasis on protection from predation suggests a change in focus for Bowlby, who in his earlier work thought of the function of attachment primarily in terms of healthy adult social behaviour, itself the result in part of healthy early attachment to a mothering figure (Bowlby, 1966). Despite this change of emphasis it is apparent that Bowlby views the mass of information on human and animal behaviour development as generally supporting his earlier view with an evolutionary justification: due to the long-standing relationship, throughout human evolution, between predation and the intensity of attachment, it is now essential to child mental health for infants to have a prolonged and close relationship in early life to a single mother or 'permanent mother-substitute.'

Before we are able to evaluate this statement in relation to the additional evidence from the study of hunter-gatherer infancy, we should examine the variety of inferences involved in making it. There is much confusion as to the ways in which reasoning from evolution really contributes to our understanding of human behaviour. At the extreme of sloppy over-confidence a series of spottily gathered facts about behaviours in various animal species which seem to exhibit analogous patterning becomes the premise for an argument of universality and evolutionary antiquity for a 'territorial imperative' (a slightly dressed-up variety of territorial instinct) (Ardrey, 1966). This is done without giving attention to numerous animal species which exhibit no territorial behaviour, or to the variability of its forms among those that do exhibit it. It is done without distinguishing between animals closely and distantly related to man or recognizing the fact that those closest to man exhibit little or no territorial behaviour. It is done without examining the range of human societies, or giving attention to the effects of subsistence ecology on such behaviour, or even glancing at the appropriate facts about man's behaviour in situations where no territoriality is evident (e.g., a hunting-gathering environment). Among the purported applications of this slenderly based 'imperative' is a presumed explanation for the failure of one phase of collectivization of agriculture in the Soviet Union. A moment's thought (or a knowledge of Russian farm economics) can supply more conventional and better reasons, and we gain nothing from such confused resort to an evolutionary account. The sort of explanation that *can* be useful should:

(1) distinguish between arguments based on phylogeny — descent from a common ancestor in the recent evolutionary past — and those based on convergent evolution — the evolution of similar behaviour (perhaps in distantly related species) because of similar selection pressures. Thus, studies of mother/infant attachment in Old World primates are more appropriately compared to human data than are such studies of precocial bird species. However, with such phenomena as pair-bonding or paternal care, rare in primates but characteristic of most birds, examination of comparable selective pressures may illuminate the origin of such behaviour in the human species (Trivers, 1972).

(2) consider the *variability* of behaviour (a) over a *phyletic range* respecting structure, adaptation, and ecological niche, and locating the human

position in this matrix, (b) *within each species* in, e.g., a variety of environments, (c) in relation to its *basis of flexibility* in a life span.

(3) consider, *in addition to* a behaviour's antiquity and the original selection pressures that led to it, *also* its present function and those pressures maintaining it — without dubious, nonfunctional, 'held-over-from-the-past' explanations. Accordingly, human-primate comparisons would consider the radically new selection pressures (including recent medical practices and social conditions) operating on the human genotype over the past million years, and the potential for rapid change introduced thereby. Probably, nonfunctional, 'held-over' traits will prove few and unimportant.

These questions have to be addressed separately and treated with different conceptions of behaviour change, ranging from the evolutionary through the sociological to the developmental. A demonstration of great antiquity or wide phyletic range, including man and his close relatives for a behaviour, is suggestive of its genic basis, but not of refractoriness to change — nor that a change will have dire consequences. Conversely, a behaviour restricted to man alone (for example, language) can be very permanent and essential. There is a *probabilistic* relationship between antiquity or range of a character and its biological 'imbeddedness,' but this cannot provide a solution for any given behaviour. A proper evolutionary argument can suggest a focus for research and testable predictions. Ardrey's argument is poor because it does neither; Bowlby's is good because it does both.

AN INTRODUCTION TO SAN INFANCY

Preliminary observation and testing of !Kung infants suggest several broad generalizations about *this group* of hunter-gatherer infants (for more detailed data see Konner, 1972; Lee and DeVore, 1974).

(1) Neurological examination of ten infants during the first ten days of life, in accord with the procedure devised by Prechtl (Prechtl and Beintema, 1964), reveals no major departure in the composition of their reflex repertoire as compared with that of European neonates. This does not mean that large matched samples would reveal no difference in the intensity of, for example, the Moro reflex, but simply that the Moro reflex could be elicited in a way comparable to the European pattern from the majority of infants.

(2) From the first few days of life (and continuing through at least the first year) infants are carried in a sling at the mother's side. This not only positions them vertically, but also insures continuous physical contact with the mother's body. In this context it is possible to see naturally occurring instances of certain reflexes, such as placing, stepping, and crawling responses

in the legs, use of the arms to move and free the head, and the grasping response. By these adjustments the infant accommodates to the mother's movements and may prevent himself smothering against her skin and clothing. Equally important, these reflexive movements serve as signals of the infant's state changes, making it possible for the mother to learn to anticipate waking, hunger, or defecation.

(3) Indulgence by the mother of the infant's dependent behaviour throughout the first year is absolute, and in the second year it slacks off only slightly. Nursing can best be described as continual, occurring over and over again throughout the day on a demand basis, and any slightly fretful signs may be interpreted as hunger signals. (It is as if the burden is on the infant to tell the mother when he is not hungry, by extruding the nipple, rather than when he is, by crying). Urination or defecation on the mother or on her clothing is met with no response during the early months except for moving and cleaning the infant after the elimination is completed. Intense physical proximity throughout the first two years makes possible a much more fine-grained responsiveness on the part of the mother with respect to the infant's needs than can be attained in a situation where the mother and infant are frequently separated by considerable distance. For example, during the first year the average amount of time elapsed (based on the data in timed, coded observations) between the onset of an infant's fretting and the mother's nurturant response was about six seconds.

(4) When not asleep or in the sling, infants are typically held sitting in the lap of the mother or another adult or child, with whom they interact in close face-to-face exchanges, or whom they use as a base for interaction with other people in the immediate vicinity. (Thanks to the subsistence ecology and the resulting structure of the band, other people are almost always available.) The frequent nursing bouts are not, in observable terms, passive events connected only with the satiation of hunger, but active behaviours in which, increasingly as the infant grows, the time, setting, choice of breast and length of the nursing session are managed entirely by the infant. This continues to be true until the time of weaning, usually during the third or fourth year. Nursing often occurs simultaneously with active play with the free breast, languid extension-flexion movements in the arms and legs, mutual vocalization, face-to-face interaction (the breasts are quite long and flexible), and various forms of self-touching, including occasional masturbation.

(5) The process of separation is initiated and carried forward almost entirely by the infant. The mother almost never leaves the infant's immediate vicinity until the later part of the second year, and then rarely until the birth of her next, usually during the fourth year. However, the infant begins to move away from the mother as soon as it is mobile, using the mother, who

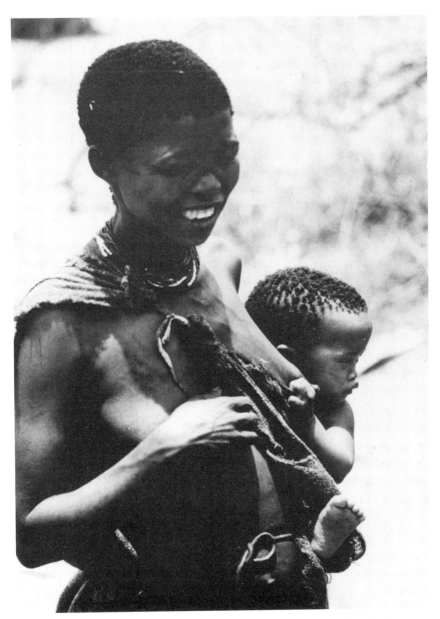

FIGURE 8 Baby and an over-the-shoulder garment cum receptacle called a *kaross* (photo: Irven DeVore)

remains sitting in the same spot, as a base for exploration. Although the prospect of becoming lost in the bush is extremely dangerous, this is very rare and is prevented both by the infant's consistent return to the mother and by the intensity of fearfulness of strangers and strange situations — an intensity much stronger than that observed in western infants (Konner, 1972). Again, because of the subsistence ecology and the nature of the band, there is usually a dense network of possible relations with children of all ages; the infant passes fairly gradually from an intense attachment to the mother, to the receptive context of a group of children — children who range in age from near-peers to adolescent caretakers, with whom the infant is both familiar and safe.

(6) The process of weaning from the breast begins at the time the mother becomes aware she is pregnant again, usually early in the third year, and weaning from being carried (which means the child, until old enough to keep up with the mother, will cease to accompany her on her gathering rounds) occurs at the time of her delivery. While neither of these processes is very abrupt or very punitive, both are relatively firm and often result in an extended period of depressed and fretful behaviour. However, there remains the consolation of the constantly present and accepting group of children which, within about a year of the infant's weaning from being carried, becomes a major focus of the latter's social behaviour.

(7) The learning of subsistence-related behaviours begins in the first year. By fifteen months of age infants are playing frequently at digging with a stick — the essential behaviour in gathering — and at chasing and striking dogs, insects, and other available living things, including people (hitting people is laughed off and not discouraged) — all essential behaviours in hunting. Particularly in the case of behaviours involved in gathering, it seems clear that infants are modelling their behaviour upon behaviours observed in their mothers, fathers, other adults, and other children.

DISCUSSION

At this stage of our knowledge it is proper to be very cautious in interpreting results, but some intimations as to the possible significance of this material can be suggested. The !Kung are not simply 'just another' non-literate society with curious and puzzling patterns of infant care among many other curious and puzzling customs. They are a hunting-and-gathering people living in a warm climate and, consequently, are constrained and guided by the pattern of subsistence ecology that was common to all human groups for roughly 99 per cent of man's time on earth. Their social organization and behaviour undoubtedly reflect better, in most respects, the situation that Bowlby calls

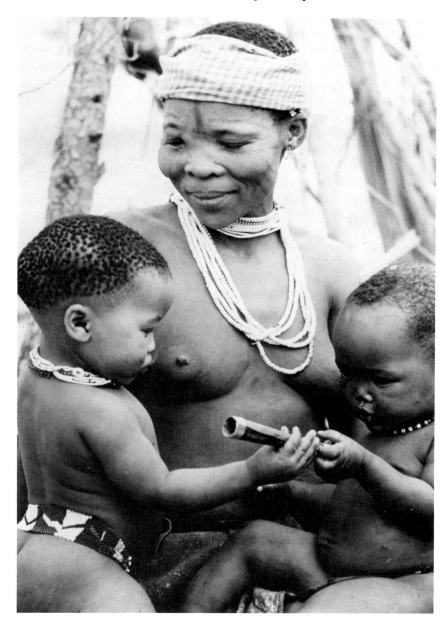

FIGURE 9 First lessons in peer relations (photo: Irven DeVore)

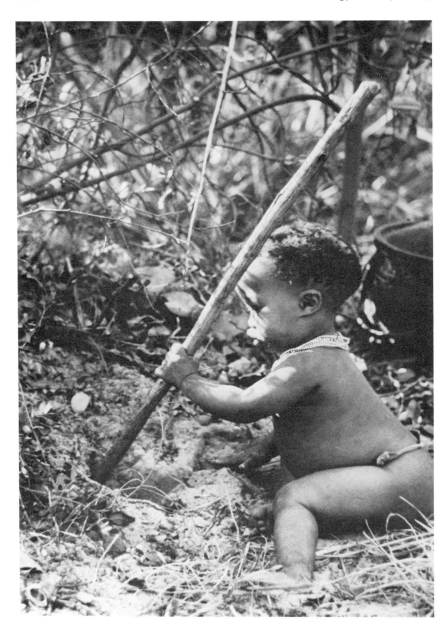

FIGURE 10 Some day this will be a way to get food (photo: Irven DeVore)

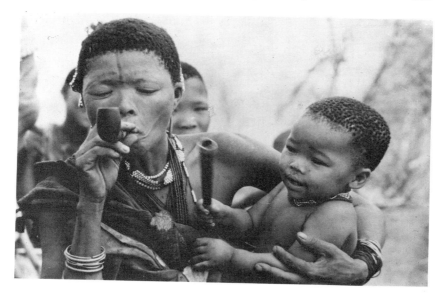

FIGURE 11   Infants are introduced early to other adults (photo: Irven DeVore)

man's 'environment of evolutionary adaptedness' than any other non-literate society for which we have good information about infant care.

The apparent implications for Bowlby's formulation and for the problems with which he is concerned are as follows:

(1) The stress on early attachment to a nurturant caretaking figure, common to Bowlby (works cited), Freud (1920), Erikson (1953), and others, is a suitable one. If anything, this position is strengthened by the facts about !Kung infancy, which reveal a mother-infant relation considerably closer, more delicately responsive, and more nurturant than the western pattern. It is also a relationship which begins relying on proximal mechanisms in attachment at birth rather than, as Bowlby suggests, in the second half year.

It must be stressed again that the importance of these data and their meaning for Bowlby's theory do not rest merely on finding similar events in a very foreign culture. The San are not merely *different* from us, they are representative of the way of life in which man and human mother/infant relations evolved. They thus stand in relation to us in a social evolutionary sequence, so that the data give mother/infant relations an historical dimension. By looking at the changes that have taken place in the mother/infant bond during the course of social evolution, we can begin to discover the antecedents and consequences of the changes.

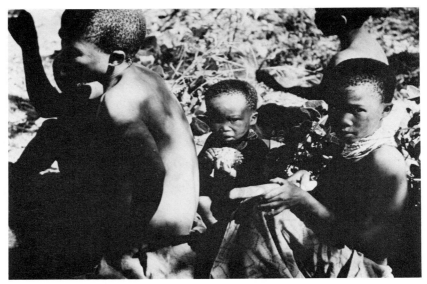

FIGURE 12   Informal affairs of the day do not interrupt contact with the children
(photo: Irven DeVore)

In the latest edition of *Baby and Child Care* Spock (1968) advises mothers to become suspicious of possible 'spoiling' of babies by the age of three months, to exercise 'a little hardening of the heart,' and if, by five or six months, the baby still expects to be picked up every time he cries, advises the mother to follow a program of 'unspoiling,' including pretending she is busy when she really is not in order to 'impress the baby' with the impossibility of responding to his fretfulness. In an apparent reversal of his position in earlier editions, Spock thus encourages the tendency of American mothers to begin shaping self-reliance in the early months of life. His advice would be viewed by Zun/wasi mothers with some combination of shock, amusement, and contempt.

However, the socio-ecological circumstances of the San must be taken carefully into account in the comparison. An American mother is not surrounded by a network of relatives and friends who can help absorb some of the practical and, even more, the emotional burdens of baby care. More important, perhaps, her child is not surrounded by a network of continuously available children of all ages who will provide an attractive alternative to attachment to the mother when the need for separation inexorably arises. In other words, the dangers of 'spoiling' may indeed be greater given the socio-ecological context of American baby care of recent decades. However, in an age of accelerating social change one need not consider the socio-ecology an absolute constant.

(2) While the data do not provide direct support for the notion of secondary drive as a process in the growth of attachment, one cannot but be impressed with the increasingly social complexion of the San nursing sessions as the infant grows through the first year, and by the whole web of attachment behaviours which occurs in the context of nursing (although they occur outside it as well). Bowlby's 'ethological' conception, that there is an innate complex of behaviours strongly predisposing the infant to attach itself to an appropriately nurturant caretaking figure, is powerfully supported by observations of growth of attachment in San (!Kung) babies. But there is no evidence to support the notion that secondary drive does not contribute at all. It is amply demonstrated in the laboratory that habits in a wide variety of animals may be strengthened by reinforcing them with the satiation of hunger. In so far as the behaviour patterns of attachment are habits, or even in the unlikely event that they are strictly innate responses, it is probable that they can be strengthened by association with the experience of hunger satiation.

(3) The observational evidence from a group of people living in man's 'environment of evolutionary adaptedness' suggests that the danger to infants of death by predation and exposure is only one part of a complex of selective forces favouring attachment during the course of evolution. If, for example, it proved to be a general law of animals with complex central nervous systems that inadequate mothering produces individuals who become abusive mothers (as Harlow, 1962, and Harlow and Harlow, 1969, found for rhesus monkeys, under admittedly severe experimental conditions), this law would result in a selection pressure as severe or more severe than any resulting from predation. Furthermore, Bowlby's earlier emphasis on attachment as a necessary base for adult social behaviour is not the mere sentimental inclination of a psychoanalyst. This function of attachment would, if valid, give it as strong an advantage in evolution as many advantageous physical characters. Adequate social behaviour is as essential to survival and reproduction as physical well-being. Finally, observational data on San (!Kung) infants support the view that adequate subsistence behaviour essential to adult survival is acquired beginning in infancy, and that it is made possible by proximity to adult models which, in turn, depends on attachment.

(4) While in the !Kung context infants are cared for almost exclusively by their mothers during the first year of life, this fact can be seen to depend upon certain aspects of the San socio-ecology. Good nutrition for the infant and protection from gastro-intestinal and other disease (a danger manifestly much greater than that of predation) requires extended and continual nursing

and an even maintenance of temperature and state. There is no nutritional substitute for milk, and the danger of gastric upset, chills, and other possible preludes to infant disease must be reduced to a minimum. The likelihood that, in a small nomadic band, there will be a woman other than the mother with freely flowing milk and no infant of her own to nurse, and who might participate significantly in the infant's care, is nil. While the San fathers play with their infants frequently and certainly are inclined toward infant nurturance, their possibilities are limited by the fact that they have no breasts. For these reasons it is easy to see why attachment to the mother exclusively (or, in rare instances, to a 'permanent mother-substitute') is unavoidable in the San adaptive context.

However, there are many other societies of ethnographic record which, under different conditions of socio-ecology, are able to provide a variety of forms of multiple-mothering or multiple-caretaking. As Margaret Mead has pointed out in a cogent critique of Bowlby's position (1966), many studies of multiple-caretaking, from traditional polygynous cultures to modern Israeli kibbutzim have failed to show that multiple-caretaking has any objectively detectable unfortunate sequelae *whatsoever*, provided that the two or three or several caretakers offer an adequately nurturant and uninterrupted human environment. The same conclusion was drawn more recently in a major review of cross-cultural studies of child development (Levine, 1970). Finally, in societies where the risk of infant death is slender, there is no evidence of ultimate biological advantage in leaving infant care exclusively to women. In so far as the mother has been pregnant for several months by the time of birth, in so far as the father can never be entirely sure that his offspring are really biologically his own, and in so far as there are still certain advantages to nursing, mothers and infants (compared to fathers and infants) will be more disposed toward each other. But that in individual cases it would be detrimental to the infant's psychological health and growth for a man and woman to participate equally – or even in a proportion favouring the man – in the care of an infant, has never been supported with reliable evidence.

It will be noted that while we have argued that some aspects of the San adaptive complex, like indulgent mothering, may well prove to be important and refractory to change without serious consequences, we have argued that another aspect, the single mother, may not. Because no data have as yet shown serious consequences of multiple parenting, we have looked for adaptive facts bearing on the need for the single mother in the evolutionary context and found them neither permanent nor compelling. On the contrary, although the natural mother is the primary caretaker, her relationship to the infant is embedded in a social network which provides important support for her. Fathers and women other than the mother absorb minor aspects of the

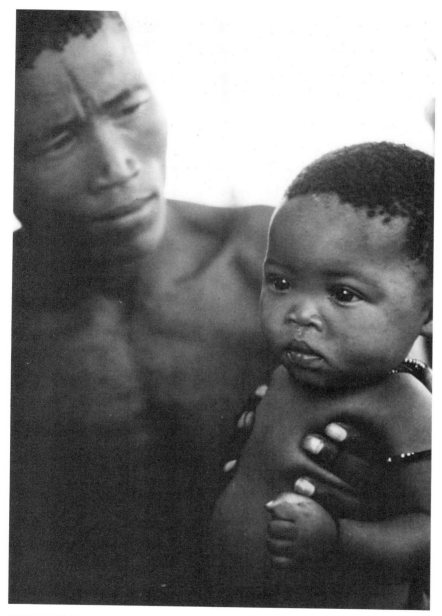

FIGURE 13 Fathers play with their infants, but have a secondary tending role (photo: Irven DeVore)

infant's care for the first year, and, thereafter, major aspects of its care and attention will fall to a multi-aged group of older children. However, a proper evolutionary argument must recognize that the antiquity of single-mothering is very great, that it is common to all of man's close relatives, and that it is present in human hunter-gatherers. This seems reason enough to continue carefully examining the consequences of multiple parenting before concluding there are no important ones. Much more research is needed.

CONCLUSIONS

We have argued that any view of the evolution of infancy, indeed, any view of human infancy at all, is incomplete without some information concerning infancy in man's 'environment of evolutionary adaptedness.' That is, only the socio-ecological conditions pertaining in hunting-and-gathering societies in warm climates can tell us what, in evolutionary terms, human infancy was meant to do and be. The San of the Kalahari Desert are only one segment of the world range of such societies, but there is ample reason to believe they are representative of this range. Furthermore they are the only such group for whom detailed information on infancy is available at this time.

Preliminary assessment of the results of this study of infancy make possible a partial evaluation of the major theoretical formulation in the area of evolution of mother infant relations, Bowlby's *Attachment*, in relation to hunter-gatherer infancy. The general emphasis on a prolonged, nurturant relationship with a mothering figure is certainly appropriate. The inborn predisposition toward attachment behaviour which Bowlby sees in the infant is certainly there. This predisposition is easily seen in San (!Kung) infants, who are carried in a sling at the mother's side from birth. But it seems that there is good reason at this time to believe that reinforcement of attachment behaviours through the satiation of hunger, warmth, and other primary reinforcers, plays some role. In addition to the dangers of predation and exposure favouring attachment behaviour through natural selection, several other selective advantages of comparable importance, obvious in the !Kung San context, are considered. Finally, while certain constraints of this context favour infant care by a single mother or permanent mother-substitute, there is no reason to suspect that in a different adaptive context adequate nurturance by several consistently present caretakers or by males is in any way detrimental.

With regard to the western world's largest selling manual of baby care (Spock, 1968), the data suggest that the difficult task of extinguishing some of these innately programmed attachment behaviours, as advised therein, is a fairly recent innovation in the evolutionary history of baby care. It seems to be related to an extreme version of certain forms of self-reliance demanded by western socio-ecology, and to the absence of a continuously present group of children of all ages in the environment of the baby to whom the latter can transfer his attachment and other social behaviours at the age of two or three, which presents the risk of a detrimentally prolonged or intense attachment to a single mothering figure. This failure of separation could probably occur only where the nuclear family is ecologically isolated, as it is in western society, and on this basis we would be inclined to predict low indulgence of attachment behaviour in early life in other societies where the mother/infant pair has only meagre social resources. Conversely, if such resources were to increase, as is possible in view of current experimentation with forms of day care and communal living, it might be possible, if judged desirable, to return to more indulgent forms of care in early life. In fact, one might predict that this will happen rather automatically, as a result of the pressure of babies upon mothers, through their inborn repertoire of attachment behaviours, evolved during more than forty million years of primate evolution.[2]

2   This has been shown by Whiting (1961). Also, prediction of low indulgence with only meagre social resources was directly addressed by a study by Rafael (1971) who showed that among urban mothers who attempt to breast-feed their infants, failure of milk-flow is most likely to occur in those mothers with the least contact with relatives, friends, and neighbours. Furthermore, intervention by a supportive, friendly (female) 'social worker' (the experimenter), shortly after failure of milk-flow caused the mother to switch to bottle-feeding, resulted in resumption of milk-flow in the majority of cases. This convincing evidence of the importance of the 'embeddedness' of the mother/infant pair in a social network shows that this factor can influence not only the sociology but also the physiology of mother/infant relations

JOHN HURRELL CROOK

7 Social Organization and the Developmental Environment

INTRODUCTION

Experimental research by a number of workers (Harlow and Harlow, 1962; Hinde et al., 1967; Mason, 1965; etc.) has already demonstrated that the social dimension has as much significance for the development of behaviour in young primates as does the physical or ecological aspect of the environment. Indeed, the crippling effects of various types of social deprivation on the development of the affective behaviour involved in reproduction and care-giving indicate that a major adaptive advantage lies with those individuals that can adjust well to their social circumstances and breed effectively within them. The relationship between the constraints set upon adaptibility by the range of social variation in the containing group, on the one hand, and the limited flexibility of the organism, on the other, is the subject of this report. At the present time the nature of our research material precludes any grand conclusions and the whole area lies wide open for study.

The relationship between the behaviour of the individual and the social organization of groups has been surprisingly neglected by ethologists. In spite of early contributions by Espinas (1878), Petrucci (1906), and Julian Huxley (1923), the mainstream of ethology has focused upon the communication and motivation of individuals usually in dyadic interaction rather than upon the group process as such (see Crook, 1970a). This means that the approach presented here has been underemphasized. The excitement of our viewpoint lies in the fact that in relation to comparisons between non-human and human primates the modern social ethology of groups is likely to break new ground worthy of close attention by anthropologists, sociologists, and psychologists alike.

THE DIVERSITY OF PRIMATE SOCIAL ORGANIZATIONS

The information which determines the development of an individual's behaviour comes from a number of different sources. Some is a consequence of the species' genetic constitution and some stems from specific relations between an individual and its mother both in the womb and post-natally. Yet further information comes from the idiosyncratic nature of individual 'trainers' such as mothers or 'aunts' who program the developing animal in mildly deviant ways. Moreover, there may be traumatic and destructive events that damage the development and produce markedly abnormal effects. There are, however, yet other factors that need consideration. For example an individual not only associates with its mother but is reared in a particular kind of social unit containing a restricted set of other companions. This social unit, as often as not, appears especially significant since it may well be the optimum social environment for child-rearing in the habitat of that particular species (Crook, 1970b). Within the unit the infant is progressively exposed to individuals in addition to the mother. Whom these may be — of what age and of what sex — is a direct consequence of the group structure and composition. Furthermore, within each group type there are highly specific sources of competitive interaction between the members. These occasion agonistic encounters that are likely to punch, hurt, or even harm the young individual. His behaviour is thus likely to be moulded to a considerable degree by the patterns of conformity he adopts in relation to his companions. Given differing group types and differing processes of social interaction within them it is hardly surprising to find that individuals of highly contrasting temperament are found in different social organizations. These differences are by no means adequately attributed to simple genetic contrasts between local populations even though these undoubtedly occur and do contribute to behavioural differentiation. The process of behaviour 'shaping' by patterns of social interaction and consequent learning — nature's Skinner Box, one might say — is a powerful source of behavioural differentiation. Where the factors are common over large populations they may produce more or less species-specific effects.

While the behaviour of an individual may be conceived as being largely a function of the patterned social interactions it encounters within the group into which it is born, the group itself may be seen as a functional interface between the traditional group-maintaining behaviour of the individual and the success with which its members feed themselves and rear young. Indeed, the social group as an environment is seen as that combination of individuals within which it is most adaptive for members of a population to disperse themselves. Although long-term ecological stability will induce traditional ways of behaving that impose constraints upon the lability of social structure, changing environments will tend to induce changes in the social organizations within which individuals live. Indeed one of the main problems in this area of research is the marked contrast in the lability of social structure shown by different species. Thus while macaques live in multimale reproductive units, and patas monkeys in one-male units with peripheral bachelor groups, the langur (*Presbytis entellus*) may occur in both of these ways – even in the same locality.

A broad survey of the social organizations of primates (Crook and Gartlan, 1966) showed that the population units or demes of these animals vary greatly in both their spatial dispersion and their composition into social units of various types. In general the primates range from small largely insectivorous lemurs and lorises which tend to be nocturnal and somewhat solitary, through diurnal forest-living and fruit-consuming monkeys living in small territorial units bossed by one or several males, to large congregations, often consisting of several structural tiers, based either upon one-male or multimale reproductive units. The latter organizations occur among the more terrestrial and open country animals. Among the great apes, the chimpanzees especially, a more open, less hierarchically organized structure appears to exist. At the time of writing most is known of social organization in the Cercopithecoidea – the Old World monkeys. These are, in any case, of special interest in relation to man since their adaptive radiation in forests and open terrain may have paralleled in important ways the pattern of radiation followed by man's immediate protohominid ancestors (Jolly, 1969). Upon these animals, therefore, we will focus our particular attention.

Table I depicts the main characteristics of the three main kinds of society shown by Cercopithecoid species. Type I shows the greatest variation in subtypes and is the most frequent kind of structure found in these animals. Clearly it must have adaptive value for its members in a wide range of habitats even though these habitats may themselves determine the variability in the spatial dispersion of the social units in the subtypical forms. It has been argued (Crook and Gartlan, 1966; Crook, 1970) that the one-male reproductive unit is the most efficient group in which to rear young in a wide diversity of circumstances. In forests where a high population density matches rich but not invarying food supplies it appears likely that a balance between numbers and resources is established at some asymptote and that the recruitment of new young to the population must approximately balance mortality unless food shortage is to occur. Territorial reservation of an exclusive range evidently secures adequate forage and the exclusion of all but one reproductive male has the effect of eliminating much intersexual competition for food. It also releases the male from much intragroup disputation over females, although it also increases his burden of territorial defence. The male possesses not only a feeding range for himself and his females but also the wherewithal for the females to rear his own young in a stable social group. The females probably 'adopt' a male who can effectively provide for themselves and for

TABLE I Some contrasting features of Cercopithecoid societies

	Type I	Type II	Type III
Social units	One-male groups Excess males	Multimale groups	Multimale groups, one-male groups, excess males
Dispersion	(1) Territorial one-male groups, e.g., *C. mitis* (2) One-male groups and all-male groups in large home ranges, e.g., *E. patas* (3) One-male groups and all-male groups in herds or moving separately, e.g., *T. gelada* (4) Excess males around periphery of band made up of one-male groups, e.g., *P. hamadryas*	In cover or areas of danger compact groups with some degree of male protection. In open areas of good visibility some tendency to scatter. Cohesion of groups seems to vary with location. E.g., *Macaca* spp., *Papio anubis*, etc.	The occurrence of the units varies with local ecology in the species range. Some areas have only multimale troops, some have all three types of unit. E.g., *Presbytis entellus*, *Colobus sp.*
Mating	Largely restricted to within the one-male groups. Some evidence of long term bonding in certain species, e.g., *P. hamadryas*. Extent of bonding probably variable between species	Mating within the multimale troop. Male access to females at time of ovulation largely a function of male dominance. Males and females consort to varying degrees at the time of mating forming rather short-term bonds at this time	Mating occurs within the local reproductive unit. In *P. entellus* certain local populations show a high degree of aggressive turnover of male ownership of one-male units. New owner, after driving out male, has been seen to kill young and mate females anew. Such behaviour is probably contingent on highly particular ecological and demographic conditions

their young. Although in theory this is attractive there remains much to work out. Aldrich-Blake (1970b) and Crook (1970) discuss the relations between spatial defensibility and food requirements. There must, it seems, balance out at some point where the animals obtain adequate resources for minimum time and energy expenditure. Where food is superabundant the maintenance of a strict territorialism appears no longer to be maintained and polyspecific groups tend to form. These appear to allow an increased protection from predation from forest eagles that take young monkeys (Gautier and Gautier-Hion, 1969; Aldrich Blake, 1970b; Gartlan, 1970).

In open country food resources tend to be patchy in both time and space as a consequence of a greater climatic variation between the seasons. Under these conditions in Africa the foraging ranges of groups must be increased to cover an adequate food supply. They thereby become increasingly difficult and eventually impossible to defend. The Patas monkeys range over vast areas as Hall (1966) showed, but maintain their social organization of one-male reproductive units. Additional males occur in 'all-male' parties that usually roam separately. Under conditions of water shortage, however, both types of group assemble together near wells and even non-reproductive group males may assist in the protection of young from predators (Struhsaker and Gartlan, 1970).

In Ethiopia the hamadryas and gelada baboons live under arid conditions, the former in the dry country of the Danakil desert and the Awash valley and the latter in the cooler montane regions with seasonal relief in the two rainy seasons. The gelada sleeps at night on the cliffs of gorges or on the crags of mountain tops. Under rich feeding conditions herds made up of harem groups and all-male groups feed in large assemblages of up to about 400 strong. Under dry-season conditions the individual groups tend to wander separately to find the patchy food. Hamadryas one-male groups tend to disperse less under poor conditions and usually remain in bands. These assemble in limited rocky sleeping sites at night. Neither geladas nor hamadryas show territoriality – they range too widely for that. Their life is based on dispersal from sleeping sites and wandering over wide ranges.

The multimale type of social structure is found in some forest species but more especially in forest fringe and woodland savannah baboons and macaques. It seems that in these habitats food is sufficiently plentiful to support a large cohesive social unit as it forages over its range. In addition, such environments often contain many potential predators and the co-operation of males in protecting the group is correspondingly advantageous. In troops of this kind there tends to be a complex dominance hierarchy based on friendships and kinship. The senior and higher status males obtain access most readily to females when the latter are in oestrus. In all kinds of social

structure, competition between males for females appears primarily responsible for the marked dimorphism in size and for differences in other characteristics between the sexes. It also plays a not unimportant role in the
stabilizing of particular grouping patterns in the different environments
(Crook, 1970).

DEVELOPMENT OF INDIVIDUAL BEHAVIOUR
IN DIFFERENT TYPES OF GROUP

Given that grouping tendencies and group composition differ in ways that are
related to ecological conditions, it is not surprising to find that the social
factors influencing infant or juvenile behaviour also differ. Indications of
these effects are provided by comparisons between mother/infant relations in
captive and wild groups. Mason (1965) has shown that for up to the first
eighteen months infant rhesus monkeys born and raised in the wild differ in
grooming behaviour, agonistic behaviour, and stability of relationships
formed between individuals, from measures of comparable behaviours in cage-
raised young. Likewise mother chimpanzees appear to interact more with
their infants in captivity than they do in the wild. Experimentally deprived
rhesus mothers treat their babies so badly that the latter may have to be hand
reared. Even short periods of experimental maternal deprivation have effects
on infant behaviour that last long after the mother's return. Clearly the
exact spacing and pattern of adult relations in wild groups must have much to
do with the emergence of individual behavioural performance and influence
the young in characteristic ways. As yet precise field studies are lacking.

Contrasts in spacing between one-male groups doubtless has much to do
with the differing adult response patterns of patas, geladas, and hamadryas
baboons in spite of similarities in their social structures. Hall (1966) and Hall
and Mayer (1967) relate the socially withdrawn character of the male patas
monkey to the dispersed character of the groups and to the males' role as
watchdog. In these groups the females are organized into hierarchies, and
females in co-operation can dominate the male. Young males are probably
ejected from the group at puberty and serve time in an all-male group elsewhere. The manner in which a young male is ejected by the reigning adult
may be determined more by female selection than by the older male's choice.

In hamadryas troops, infant males and females often seek the protection
of a juvenile or sub-adult male who may then threaten their pursuer. These
males in fact play the role of substitute mothers (Kummer, 1967) albeit
somewhat capricious ones. When juvenile males reach the age of two years
they are no longer protected in this way and drift into the all-male section of
the band. Young females are however still cared for, usually by particular

males, of whose harems they eventually form the nucleus. Sub-adult males may also gradually acquire a harem by teaming up with an older harem owner. As the latter ages the younger animal gradually 'inherits' the females, even though the direction of march is usually determined by the older male who is carefully watched by the younger one. These types of behaviour involve complex social skills. The young male who learns to retain younger females by solicitous care, or the one who placates an old male sufficiently to remain teamed with him, are both intelligent manipulators of the social scene whose work earns them rewards in terms of female reproductives and the consequent offspring. The conditioning process here is clearly complex and in part a function of the kind of social structure in which the animals occur. In the gelada, the rather more dispersed pattern of environmental exploitation in the dry season may perhaps be a factor preventing the acquisition of females through protection and mothering. At any rate in these animals, while two-male teams are known, the 'maternal' method of acquiring a young female has yet to be recorded.

In multimale groups the pattern of maternal interaction with babies differs in contrasting species. Baboon and rhesus macaque mothers are generally firmly attached to their babies and resist separation. Langur mothers, at least in Jay's (1965) study area, permit 'aunts' to hold and carry infants soon after birth. In captivity rhesus mothers may also permit this (Rowell et al., 1964) while in Barbary macaques the baby seems to be almost perpetually circulating among interested young males and 'aunts' alike, often for long periods of time before it returns to its mother (Deag and Crook, 1971; Burton, 1971). Young males of this species in the Middle Atlas mountains were found to take babies from mothers or aunts and look after them carefully. Often this behaviour was associated with the presentation of the baby to older males. It appears that this behaviour in some way regulates the probability of antagonism between males. As in certain other species, if a fight breaks out a male may grab a baby and achieve immunity from severe attack by so doing. Deag and Crook (1971) have suggested that a kind of 'agonistic buffering' appears to be going on.

A comparable activity has been reported by Itani (1959) in three out of eighteen Japanese macaque troops. Here one-year-old juveniles were adopted by males when the mothers gave birth to new young. In one case a male was known to rise in social status as a result and Itani suggested that affiliation with the young of high status troop members might improve the rank of the performer. The local occurrence of this activity suggests it to be a proto-cultural phenomenon limited to certain troops only.

Vandenberg (1967) reported that when small troops of rhesus monkeys were introduced on to small islands off Puerto Rico the most stable social element comprised the adult females. The presence of a dominant male was, however, essential for group maintenance. The social organization of these populations was unstable, a fact that Vandenberg attributed to the absence of long-term matrilineal kinship relations between the introduced animals. The effect of behavioural maturation within such a network of affiliations is certainly of great importance for later behavioural performance and the acquisition of relatively high status in the troop. A high status animal is characterized by relatively 'high profile' behaviour, an assertive manner, confident posture and gait, and willingness to be aggressive. Low status animals by contrast are nervous, move hesitatingly with much avoidance of others, and flee easily when they are threatened. Their low profile performance is likely to be associated with some degree of physiological stress. Whether or not the life trajectory of an individual involves high or low status, behaviour must be largely determined by the pattern of relations among its immediate kin and also by its own personal success-to-failure ratio in agonistic competition with peers. Wilson (1969) showed that among the feral rhesus monkeys on Cayo Santiago island there is a considerable movement of young males from one group into the all-male periphery of another. The transfer is not always easy and a would-be entrant often gains a 'sponsor' which turns out to be a close relative from the natal troop – probably a brother. Affiliations between males in all-male groups may be commonly based upon friendships that originated in the natal group.

SOCIAL DYNAMICS IN MULTIMALE GROUPS

In analyses of multimale groups of baboons and macaques similar social structure is found again and again. There is usually a dominant alpha or 'control' male operating in the behavioural control of other members through the aid given him by affiliated henchmen (Hall and DeVore, 1965; Bernstein, 1966, etc.). The subordinate males and females may occupy a relatively 'peripheral' part of the troop as Japanese studies have shown. The position of an individual within this structure is not, however, necessarily fixed. His allocation to a given social position at any one time is evidently the outcome of a number of interacting processes that sort out group members into various ranked categories – which are not necessarily the same across all behavioural dimensions. Individuals are exposed to this process throughout life and the probability of high rank must relate to their success in dealing with social forces impinging on them from early in life.

Factors that bring about changes in social position are various. As young males mature they will seek with vigour to mate with females, but will tend to be prevented by older animals. As males age, by contrast, they will cease to be reproductively active, although they may retain high status positions in some cases virtually till death. Habits of deference set up in groups can be very long lasting indeed. Young males may also form friendships, however, and when a shift in the power structure occurs may operate together to change their situation. Behaviour patterns of deference give way to those of assertion: with competitive success their whole deportment and behavioural repertoire changes (see Reynolds, 1970). Females show changes in social position often in correlation with oestrus as they move in and out of consort with dominant males.

As the group increases in number, splits may occur with subgroups of affiliated animals forming branch troops. Under these circumstances males of formerly relatively low status can become the new 'control' animals. In some Japanese reports the leadership of branch troops is often unstable. In particular, an adult male who deserted the troop earlier and who has been living solitarily may abandon that manner of life and join the branch group to become its controlling member.

In general, one may say that the social dynamics of a primate social unit express the effects of two contrary forces: the individual's attempt to satisfy all its needs, and the social competition arising when commodities are either in short supply or preempted by other animals. An individual is born into such a situation and has initial advantages or disadvantages depending upon his kinship links and the affiliations he develops through association with elder relatives, peers, and care-giving males or females. The individual may also be utilized by others in 'games' of social subterfuge such as the apparent agonistic buffering process recorded in Japanese and Barbary macaques. The role sequence shown by an individual throughout his life trajectory must have a close link with these starting conditions. So far, however, we have no thoroughly studied case histories with which to analyse such a process. Particular individuals appear to try to avoid behavioural constraint, probably because of the unpleasant affect produced in social stress. As we have seen, the avoidance of constraint may be achieved in several ways including co-operative aggression associated with upward change in status, going solitary, subterfuge through skillful social manipulation of others affiliated to high ranked animals, and the assumption of assertive behaviour when the 'fission threshold' (e.g., Sugiyama, 1960; Mizuhara, 1964) in group size is reached and a split occurs. The maintenance of relatively unconstrained behaviour is aided by co-operative alliances with other assertive individuals, by the performance of a control role in breaking up quarrels which is a focus for protected threat, and in showing group care in defensive responses to predators and non-group conspecifics. It is also facilitated by the rewards others receive through the protective behaviour provided them and by the avoidance learning of submissive animals following encounter and punishment. These forces for stasis in a group are strong and probably more characteristic of a group dynamic situation than is role reversal and the breakdown of behaviour into aggression.

Cercopithecoid species differ greatly in the flexibility of their social organizations. The greatest range of group structure is shown by the Hanuman langur (Jay, 1965; Sugiyama, 1967). In some areas it lives in multimale groups, in others in all-male groups with associated one-male units. In yet other areas multimale, one-male, and all-male units all occur in the same region. The ecological explanation of the local occurrence of these contrasts remains unclear but much aggressive interaction, with repeated take-overs of female parties by males that may even kill off the existing young and then mate with their mothers, may be associated with conditions of overpopulation and habitat restriction. Nevertheless, it is clear that Colobine monkeys do show greater flexibility in social organization than do the macaques, for example, and this may be a consequence of genetic factors allowing for greater social variation. How such differences are determined remains unknown.

A little studied aspect of Cercopithecoid group life concerns the effect of sexual drive on social organization. Mating seasons are commonly limited to a few months and may or may not be associated with marked changes in the female anatomy. In particular the occurrence of sexual swellings in the ischial region may be linked with the production of pheromones functioning as a male aphrodisiac (Michael and Keverne, 1968, 1970). The reasons why some species show such swellings and why other closely related species do not remain to be elucidated. At present we do not know in what way those contrasts affect differentially the social life of the forms concerned. There is an important field here wide open for further research.

CONCLUSION

We have seen that primate social structures vary in relation to taxonomic status and in relation to ecology. They appear to be well adapted to their respective habitats and comprise dispersion and group composition patterns in which individuals of the species survive and procreate most successfully.

Evidence suggests that the differing organizations of primate groups play a considerable role in influencing the behavioural development shown by young animals. The infant is affected by both kinship and non-kin affiliative relationships, by the gender and character of adult individuals that interact with him in various ways, and by rewards and punishments encountered when in competition with others for some desired commodity. Primate social dynamics represent a working out of tensions arising from competition that inevitably constrains the behaviour of some individuals more than others. Strategies to avoid constraint involve the young in tactics of solitarization or affiliative co-operation in behaviour assertion when social circumstances permit. Babies and infants may be used by subordinate adult or sub-adult males to regulate the latter's behaviour in relation to adult dominants. The details of this form of co-operative subterfuge and baby utilization remain to be fully explored but a baby's future may well be affected by its forced or voluntary participation in such higher primate 'games.'

Many developmental studies have been concerned with detailed analyses of animals in relatively restricted circumstances. The effects on individual development of the wide diversity of higher primate societies in nature remains to be worked out. Such study necessitates long-term field programmes. In view of the human threat to so many natural habitats the sooner these are undertaken the better. There may be less time available for such work than we might like to think.

WILLIAM A. MASON

8   Differential Grouping Patterns
in Two Species
of South American Monkey*

This paper is concerned with primate grouping tendencies. Dr Crook has explained in an article in this book how primate groups may be classified into various structural types, such as the one-male group and the multimale group. He also indicates that species differ in the type of social structures they usually display. For example, the hamadryas baboon is characteristically organized in one-male groups, while the basic unit in the savanna baboons is the multimale group.

We know, of course, that social structure is a static and rather idealized concept. Social structures are not constant over time (they can vary during different stages in the history of a group) or space (different populations of the same species may show disparate patterns of social organization). In spite of this variability, however, it is clear that species do have their own characteristic organizational patterns. This poses an interesting question. Primate social systems are inherently open and variable. Yet, for any given species social systems assume a characteristic form. What is responsible for the fact that different species structure their social groups in distinct and contrasting ways?

In approaching this question it will be useful to recall Dr Crook's distinction between the structure of the group and the processes through which that structure is created and maintained. This distinction implies that different social structures are the result of different social processes. It follows that if one is interested in getting at the immediate (proximate) causes of species differences in social organization, the relations between group members is one of the first places to look. That is the general rationale for the approach described herein.

The discussion concerns two species of South American monkey that show different patterns of social organization in the wild. It is assumed that these differences are based on behavioural traits or predispositions – grouping

* This research was supported by grants GB-8202 from the National Science Foundation and FR-00164 from the National Institutes of Health

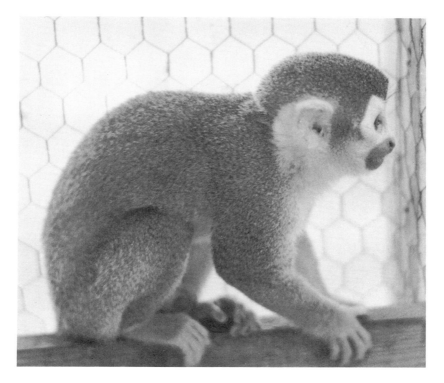

FIGURE 1 Squirrel monkey, *Saimiri sciureus*

tendencies — that can be identified and that interact with the environment to determine the structure of the social system that either species might actually display in any particular set of circumstances. The nature of these predispositions is the problem that will chiefly concern us here.

NATURAL SOCIAL ORGANIZATION OF SAIMIRI AND CALLICEBUS

First, an introduction to the monkeys, and a brief resumé of their natural history: one of the two species, the squirrel monkey (Saimiri) is probably familiar to everyone. It is the little greenish-yellow monkey that one sees so often in pet shops (Figure 1). The single field study we have on the squirrel monkey indicates that the modal pattern of social organization in this species is the multimale unit (Thorington, 1967, 1968). The group contains variable numbers of adult males, adult females, and young of both sexes in all stages of development. The squirrel monkey group ranges over a sizeable area, the boundaries of which are poorly defined. During the day the group often breaks up into clusters or subgroups which are widely dispersed, but at night the animals generally sleep together in the same group of trees.

Little is known of the relations between different groups of Saimiri. Casual reports of parties of several hundred individuals suggest that distinct groups may sometimes merge into a single large troop, but Thorington found no indication of this in his field study and systematic investigations of the relations between laboratory groups suggest that it is an unlikely possibility (Castell and Ploog, 1967; Rosenblum, Levy, and Kaufman, 1968). In any event, there is no evidence of any distinctive and recurrent pattern of inter-group meetings. Probably groups are widely enough dispersed under most conditions and their ranges are so large that they seldom come into contact and can easily avoid each other on the few occasions when they happen to meet.

The other species, the titi monkey (Callicebus), is rarely seen in captivity, even in zoos (Figure 2). It too, has been the subject of only one field study, covering an eleven-month period (Mason, 1966, 1968). We have found that, in sharp contrast to the squirrel monkey, Callicebus characteristically live in small family-type groups consisting of an adult male and an adult female who apparently remain together indefinitely, and one or two young. Each group occupies an area covering about an acre as a permanent and exclusive preserve. The younger animals leave the group as they became mature, partly because the adults begin to treat them roughly. Presumably, they eventually meet other solitary animals, form pairs, and set up new social units. Virtually nothing certain is known about the formation of new groups. The population most intensively observed lived in a small seventeen-acre savannah-surrounded grove which apparently was, from the residents' point of view, fully occupied, since newly mature animals just separated from their natal group did not establish themselves in the forest where they had grown up, but left it, probably heading out for one of the larger forests nearby. Within this grove, nine distinct groups of Callicebus could be identified. Their locations and compositions are shown in Figure 3.

The relations between adjacent groups was one of the most dramatic and distinctive features of the social life of Callicebus. Almost every day, usually in the morning, neighbouring groups met at the borders of their home ranges and engaged in an elaborate confrontation. As the groups opposed each other in trees a few yards apart, the members of a group drew close to each other; they showed conspicuous pilorection, particularly of the tail; they called vigorously and at length; they arched their backs, bowed their arms, and

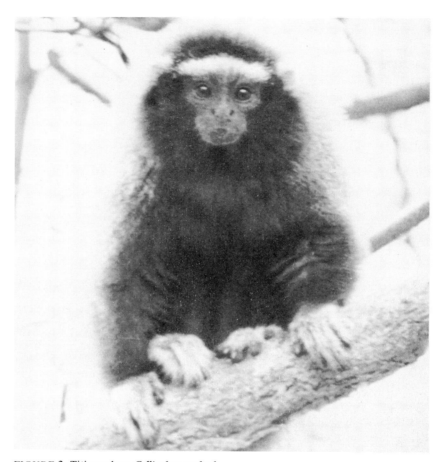

FIGURE 2 Titi monkey, *Callicebus moloch*

lashed their tails. The groups chased each other back and forth. Confrontations might last anywhere from ten minutes to a half-hour. The groups then moved apart, each returning to the core of its home area where it resumed the more pedestrian activities that made up the bulk of the daily routine — feeding, grooming each other, or just sitting quietly with tails intertwined.

Although there is little doubt that these meetings between neighbouring groups helped to maintain the home area as an exclusive preserve, the confrontation was not, strictly speaking, a form of territorial defence. There was never any indication that groups were attempting either to extend their living

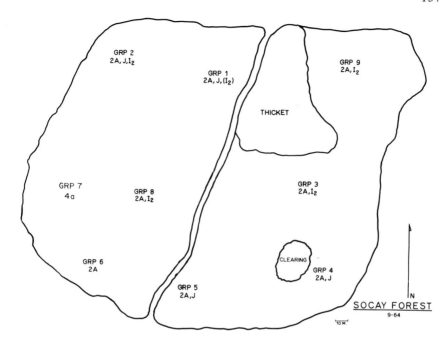

FIGURE 3 Location of titi monkey groups and group composition in primary study site. A = adult, J = juvenile or subadult, I_2 = late infant, no longer carried. Age class of animals in group 7 was uncertain (after Mason, 1966)

space or to repel invaders. In fact, the outcome of any particular confrontation had no discernible effect on the size of the territory or the location of its boundaries. On the contrary, the territories were remarkably stable over time and the confrontations occurred at definite — one could almost say 'agreed upon' — locations with predictable regularity. This is suggested in Figure 4 which shows the sites where confrontations occurred between three neighbouring groups.

Sex and parenthood also had their unusual aspects in Callicebus. During the breeding season relations between neighbouring groups followed much the same pattern as during the rest of the year, except that mating sometimes occurred between groups. These were temporary liaisons, often lasting only a few minutes, after which the wayward male and female rejoined their customary partners. After babies arrived there was an intriguing division of labour in which the male carried the infant most of the time. The mother took the baby to suckle it and clean it, and when she had finished, the baby

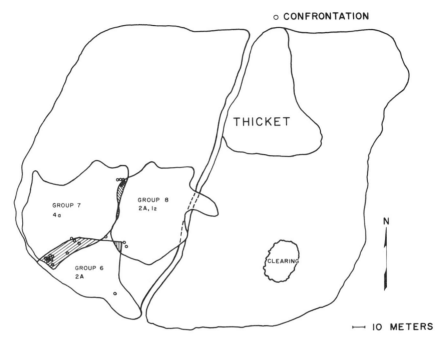

FIGURE 4 Home ranges of groups 6, 7, 8. Cross-hatching indicates overlap of group ranges. Circles indicate sites of confrontations between the three groups (after Mason, 1968)

either returned to the male under its own power — aided and abetted by the mother who usually sat close beside her mate — or the male simply lifted it off its mother's back.

These are the major features of the natural history of Saimiri and Callicebus as we know them today. The story is incomplete, to be sure, but we can be confident that the social systems of Callicebus and Saimiri differ markedly in the wild, even when these monkeys live in the same forest (Thorington, 1968). Thus, the contrasts in social organization reflect something more than a simple and direct result of differences in habitat. Each species has its own distinctive pattern of responses to the environment.

With the discontinuation of the field research, our attention was turned to the study of captive animals in the hope of getting more information about the sources of group differences in social organization. The laboratory situation has the virtue of allowing one to observe at close range the social adjustments and group reactions of different species to identical circumstances, a possibility which is rarely encountered in the wild. Furthermore, one can arrange those circumstances so as to focus on specific questions.

STUDIES ON CAPTIVE ANIMALS

Since the field observations suggested a strong and abiding affinity between male and female titi monkeys, but not between male and female Saimiri, the social bond provided an obvious starting point for our studies. Was there, indeed, a special attraction between male and female Callicebus? How strong and how specific was it?

Our first step in approaching this problem was to observe the normal behaviour of male-female pairs in the living cage. In all there were ten pairs of each species. Each pair lived and was observed in an outdoor cage, which was spacious by ordinary laboratory standards (8 by 8 by 4 ft wide). In keeping with the field data, we found evidence of greater sociability in Callicebus. Cagemates stayed closer together; they were more often in contact; and they spent more time grooming each other. Furthermore, their movements within the cage were more closely co-ordinated. For example, when we compared the total activity scores of male and female in each pair of titi monkeys we obtained a substantial correlation coefficient (rho = 0.81, $p = 0.01$), whereas the comparable value for squirrel monkeys was small and non-significant (rho = 0.21).

The amount of information that can be obtained from merely observing the normal activities of isolated pairs is quite limited in some respects, of course, and a more direct and sensitive measure of the strength and specificity of the pair bond was obviously desirable. Our approach to this problem was crude, but it turned out to be quite effective. We used a tunnel cage, twenty feet long, with a runway down the centre, terminating on either end at two small cages in which we could place other monkeys as social incentives. In one incentive cage the subject might find its cagemate, and in the other, a female stranger. The subject's position on the runway was noted at intervals of fifteen seconds during a five-minute period and these data were used to derive social preference score.

Ten males and ten females of each species were tested for twenty sessions under each of five different incentive conditions: (1) the cagemate and a female stranger; (2) the cagemate and a male stranger; (3) the cagemate and an empty incentive cage; (4) the male stranger alone; (5) the female stranger alone. In other words, two conditions allowed the animal to choose between the cagemate and a stranger of either sex, and three conditions offered a choice between a social incentive and nothing.

PREFERENCE FOR CAGEMATE

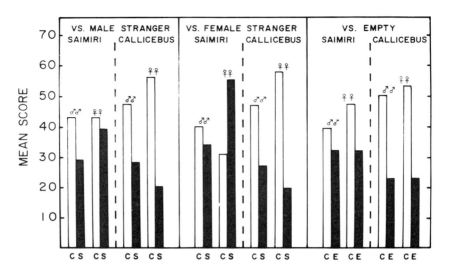

FIGURE 5 Social preference tests. Cagemate vs male stranger, female stranger and empty cage. C = cagemate, S = stranger, E = empty cage

The results were in good agreement with previous findings, but there were a few surprises, particularly from the squirrel monkeys. Figure 5 shows preference for the cagemate (C) when it was presented with a male or female stranger (S), or alone (E). In every comparison, the preference for the cagemate was stronger in Callicebus than in Saimiri ($p = 0.002$ for the combined conditions).

Callicebus of both sexes preferred the cagemate under all conditions, although the preference was most consistent in the females than in the males. All differences shown for Callicebus in Figure 5 are statistically reliable, except the male's preference for the cagemate when she was paired with a male stranger.

The pattern of preferences was more complicated in Saimiri than Callicebus since it depended upon the sex of the subject, the sex of the incentive animal, and the specific alternatives that were available. Males and females both preferred the cagemate over a male stranger, but group differences were not large for either sex, and fall short of statistical significance. In general, preferential reactions to the male were sharper among the males, and at the same time showed greater variability across individuals. Six of the ten Saimiri males showed a significant preference for the cagemate over the male stranger

PREFERENCE (VS. EMPTY)

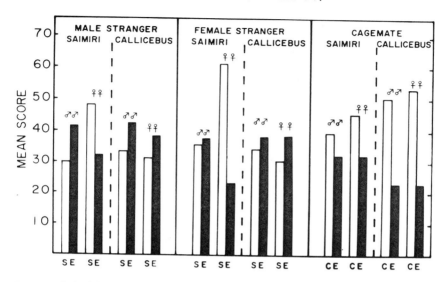

FIGURE 6 Social preference tests. Preferences for male stranger (S), female stranger (S), vs empty cage (E)

and three males showed a significant preference for the stranger. On an individual basis, only one female showed a reliable preference for the cagemate, although none showed a reliable preference for the male stranger. The condition in which the cagemate was presented with a female stranger produced the clearest and most surprising result in squirrel monkeys. As Figure 5 suggests, females overwhelmingly preferred a female stranger to their male cagemate ($p = 0.01$). As a group, the males showed a slight and non-significant preference for their cagemate over the unfamiliar female. The difference between the sexes in preference for the female stranger is highly significant ($p = 0.002$).

The three conditions in which only a single social incentive was presented (Figure 6) offer some additional information on the contrasts between sexes and species. Squirrel monkey males and titi monkeys of both sexes 'preferred' the empty cage in the presence of strangers; that is, they showed a slight (but non-significant) tendency to avoid the unfamiliar animals. Saimiri females, however, were attracted to both strangers, and, again, the attraction to the unfamiliar female was particularly strong. The preference for either stranger over the empty cage was reliable, as was the preference for the female stranger over the male ($p = 0.01$).

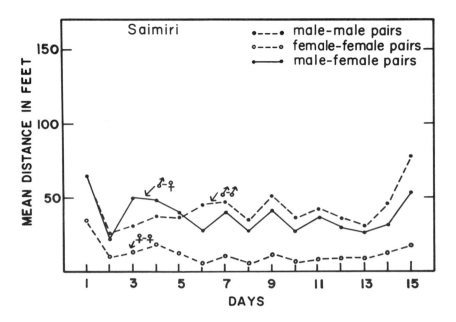

FIGURE 7 Social distance: between males, between females, and between males and females in *Saimiri* (after Mason and Epple, 1969)

Other tests have given us much the same picture. One of these is a situation which offered a good deal more scope for social interaction than any we have considered thus far. The research setting was a 100 by 400 ft outdoor enclosure, equipped with a network of runways made up of twenty-five-foot sections. Each section was identified by a number, and divided into five colour-coded segments, which enabled us quickly to determine each animal's location within the enclosure. Six shelters, each containing a supply of food and water, were evenly distributed within the enclosure (Mason and Epple, 1969).

Our procedure was to release six animals (three 'established' male-female pairs) at a time into the enclosure, where they remained undisturbed until the experiment was completed several weeks later. Every weekday for 15 days the group was observed for five hours, and at five-minute intervals throughout this period the location of each animal and the nature of its activity was recorded. The experiment was repeated with three different sex-animal groups from each species.

Consider first the findings on social distance. Distance between males, between females, and between males and females are presented for Saimiri

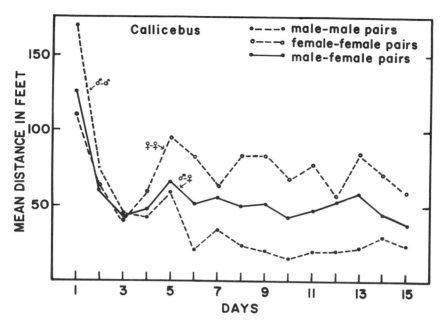

FIGURE 8 Social distance: between males, between females, and between males and females in *Callicebus* (after Mason and Epple 1969)

and Callicebus in Figures 7 and 8. Social distance was greater over all in Callicebus than in Saimiri ($p = 0.002$) and the pattern of differences by sexes was entirely consistent with results from preference testing. In the squirrel monkeys, distance was least between females, and about equal between males and between males and females, while in the titis, distance was greatest between females, intermediate between males and females, and least between males.

When we consider the effects of prior living arrangements, further contrasts between species emerge. Figure 9 shows that for titi monkeys the distance between former cagemates was substantially less than that between previously unacquainted male-female pairs ($p = 0.01$), while former squirrel monkey cagemates were not much closer to each other than to strangers of the opposite sex.

Findings on social contact are consistent with this picture (Figure 10). Contacts between former squirrel monkey cagemates were only slightly higher than contacts between previously unacquainted males and females and the difference is not statistically reliable. In Callicebus, however, former cagemates were much more often in contact than were unacquainted males and females (p = 0.01).

An analysis of specific patterns of social interaction likewise indicates that the relation between former cagemates was far more influential in Callicebus than in Saimiri. Titi monkeys more often approached and followed their cagemates than strangers of either sex (106.7 vs 67.5, p = 0.05), cagemates groomed each other more often than strangers (23.4 vs 14.6, p = 0.05), and they more often sat together with their tails intertwined (50.3 vs 24.7, p = 0.01). On each of these measures the differences were sharper for the females than for the males.

In Saimiri prior acquaintance of male and female had little apparent effect on specific patterns of social interaction. The most influential factor by far was the attraction of individuals to members of their own sex. Squirrel monkeys approached and followed like-sexed animals nearly twice as frequently as animals of the opposite sex (42.3 vs 24.5, p = 0.05); moreover, former cagemates were approached and followed only slightly more often than strangers of the opposite sex (30.5 vs 27.5).

DISCUSSION

These studies have been reviewed in detail in order to illustrate one approach to the analysis of species differences in social structure. We have found that Saimiri and Callicebus differ in the particular patterns of affinities and aversions existing between the sexes. With this information we are in a better position to describe the grouping tendencies that contribute to the characteristic types of social organization that each species displays in nature.

Of the two species, Callicebus appears to be the more conservative and exclusive in its social relations. Titi monkeys of both sexes develop an abiding affinity to familiar companions of the opposite sex – a pair bond – and both show considerable caution in approaching strangers. The sexes are not equivalent, however, and these characteristics are more prominent in the female. Her attachment to the male is stronger – or at least more exclusive – than his attachment to her.

Saimiri show an altogether different pattern. In contrast to Callicebus, it is the female squirrel monkey that appears to be the more open to new social contacts, the more persistently gregarious. And her strongest attraction, by far, is to members of her own sex. Saimiri males appear to be more cautious in their approach to novel situations than are the females. Most males prefer familiar over unfamiliar females and they avoid unfamiliar males or respond to them aggressively. When males are allowed to live together for some weeks, however, aggression drops to a very low level and most of their time is spent

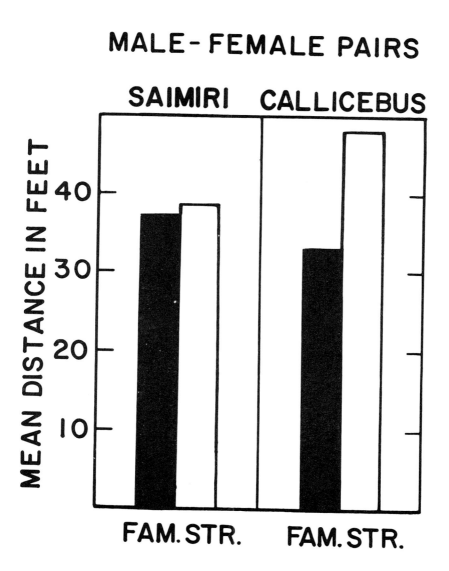

FIGURE 9 Distance between former cagemates (FAM) and previously unacquainted male-female pairs (STR) in *Saimiri* and *Callicebus* (after Mason and Epple, 1969)

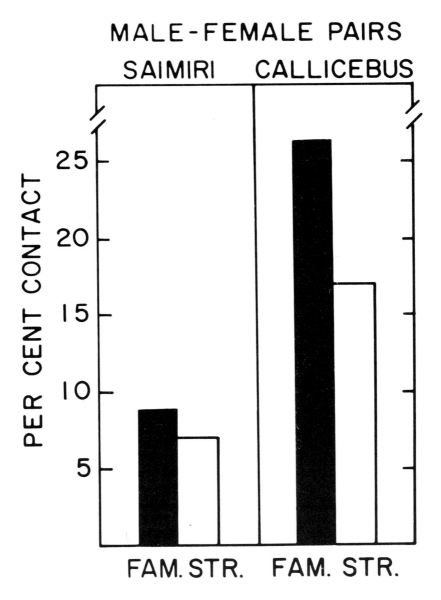

FIGURE 10 Percentage of contacts between former cagemates (FAM) and previously unacquainted male-female pairs (STR) in *Saimiri* and *Callicebus*

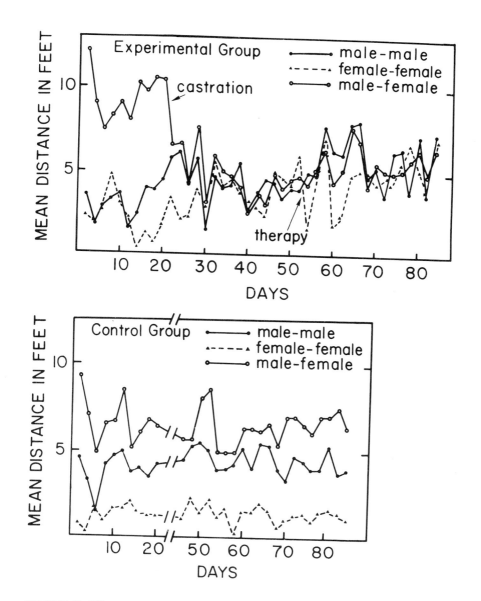

FIGURE 11 Effects of castration on mean distance between males, between females, and between males and females in *Saimiri* (after Alvarez, 1968)

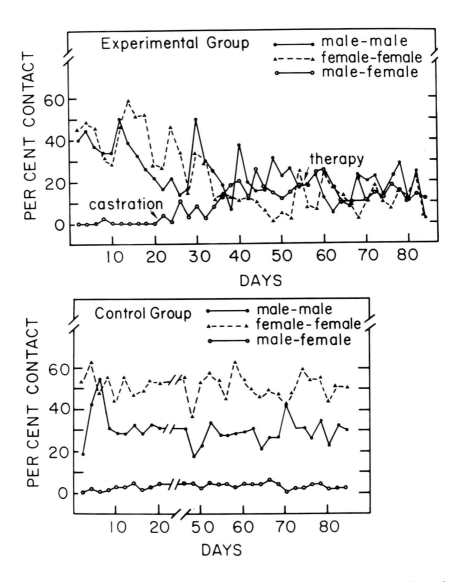

FIGURE 12 Effects of castration on contacts between males, between females, and between males and females in *Saimiri* (after Alvarez, 1968)

amiably in each other's company. Along with the males' attraction to each other, however, they are also persistently drawn to the females and form a kind of satellite or peripheral subgroup located around a more tightly clustered female nucleus.

Table I is an attempt to represent these patterns of attraction in the two species, in relation to the sexes and to familiarity.

TABLE I   Grouping tendencies

	Response to strangers	
	Male strangers	Female strangers
Saimiri		
Male	+ −	+ −
Female	+	+ + +
Callicebus		
Male	+ −	+ −
Female	−	−

	Response to familiar companions	
	Male	Female
Saimiri		
Male	+ + +	+ +
Female	+ +	+ + + +
Callicebus		
Male	+ +	+ + +
Female	+ + + +	+ −

Because of the prominence of sex differences in social organization, one might suppose that gonadal hormones are influential variables. A study conducted on squirrel monkeys by Dr Fernando Alvarez indicates that this is true (Alvarez, 1968). In this research Alvarez used two groups of squirrel monkeys, each group consisting of three males and three females. The characteristic squirrel monkey social structure was evident in each group within a few days after they were established: social distance was least and social contacts were highest between females; distance and contacts were at an intermediate level between males, and distance was greatest and contacts were least between males and females (see Figures 11 and 12). After twenty-five days all of the animals in one group were gonadectomized. Within 10 days after the group was re-established following post-surgical recovery this characteristic pattern was completely abolished. It should be noted, however, that in spite of the dramatic change in social organization following castration, hormone replacement had no discernible effect.

EVOLUTIONARY PERSPECTIVE

COLIN G. BEER

9   Comparative Ethology
and the Evolution of Behaviour

According to Lorenz (1950) comparative ethology owes its existence to the discovery that there are patterns of behaviour that can be regarded in the same way as features of anatomy. In this and many of his other comments on the evolution of behaviour, and the use of behavioural characteristics in taxonomy, Lorenz has made it apparent that ethology is heir to one of the oldest disciplines in biology: namely, comparative morphology. Comparison of the forms of animals occupied Aristotle in his zoological writings. It dominated zoological teaching and debate in the 18th and much of the 19th century. It provided Darwin with one of the major sources of evidence for his thesis that organisms have undergone evolution.

This thesis revolutionized biology, as we all know. But it is sometimes useful to recall that *The Origin of Species* (1859) contained two arguments about evolution, for their influences in biological study were to some extent distinct and can still be distinguished in the ways in which the evolution of behaviour is discussed and studied. On the one hand there was the argument that organisms are related to one another by descent with modification from common ancestors, and hence that the variety of forms of life has an historical continuity that can be pieced together by study of comparative morphology, palaeontology, biogeography, and embryology. The concept of evolution provided a unifying principle for facts from these various sources. It gave rise to a tradition in which such facts are construed historically to arrive at conclusions about lineages: from family trees or phylogenetic relationships, inferences about the ancestral origins and genealogies of species characteristics may be made. On the other hand there was the argument that the process underlying evolution is natural selection: the differential perpetuation of heritable variations as a consequence of selective agencies favouring some variations over others. One of the outcomes of natural selection is adaptation. The concept of natural selection brought new impetus and new thinking to an old subject: the appearance of design in nature. Biologists began trying to interpret or explain the characteristics of organisms in terms of their adaptive significance, and hence the selection pressures that have determined their evolutionary history and are responsible for their preservation.

In the study of the evolution of behaviour, then, one can distinguish two kinds of question (1) The historical question: from what did this or that piece of behaviour evolve, and via what intermediate stages? (2) The question of survival value: what is the adaptive significance of this or that piece of behaviour? As a consequence of what selection pressures was it evolved and is at present preserved? The kinds of evidence that bear on these two types of question are different. It is to the historical question rather than to the question of survival value that the legacy of comparative morphology has made its contribution to ethology.

Central to the discipline of comparative morphology are two closely related concepts: the concept of shared patterns of structural organization, and the concept of homology. All the animals we call vertebrates have the same plan: a backbone divided into vertebrae with a skull at one end and two pairs of limbs attached along its length. It is because these animals share this structural plan that we call them vertebrates and class them together in taxonomy as animals of the same general type. Similarly, all arthropods (animals like crayfish, insects, spiders, and so forth) have the skeleton on the outside of the body and a segmental arrangement of parts. In all groups of animals the sharing of structural organization could be thus exemplified. It is in accordance with such shared morphological patterns that animals are classified as this kind or that.

The wing of a bird, the forelimb of a frog, and the arm of a man all occupy corresponding positions in the structural plan that vertebrates share. Even within each of these different kinds of structure – the wing, the arm, and so forth – one can perceive corresponding relationships between the parts. Hence the sharing of labels such as humerus or radius for the bones. Such correspondence between the parts of two or more different types of organism that share a common structural plan is what was classically meant by structural homology.

Note that in this attempt at a definition of structural homology no reference is made to common origins, either evolutionary or genetic. The conception that structures have origins or antecedents in an evolutionary historical sense was not present in the thinking of the eighteenth-century anatomists who developed the concept of homology. The theory of evolution provided explanation for the existence of homologies. In the interests of logic it is usually important not to confuse *explicans and explicandum,* but in biology the explanation of homology has tended to usurp the meaning of the term. Homology is now usually thought of in terms of common origins (community of descent) in an evolutionary sense, and it is this kind of

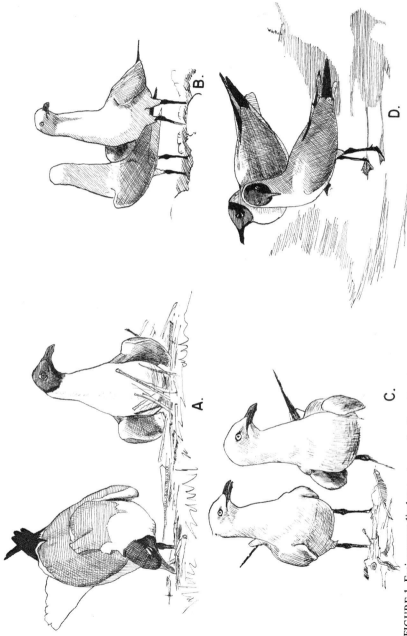

FIGURE 1 Facing-away display postures of gulls. A Laughing Gull (*Larus atricilla*); B Black-billed Gull (*Larus bulleri*); C Red-billed Gull (*Larus novaehollandiae scopulinus*); D Black-headed Gull (*Larus ridibundus*). (Drawn from photographs)

definition that you will find in most of the textbooks. Nevertheless, in the practice of comparative morphology it is still the old eighteenth century meaning of the term that provides the main criterion for recognition of structural homologies — the 'Principle of Connection' which defines homology in terms of relationship relative to shared patterns of organization.

In comparative ethology a concept of homology is just as central as in comparative morphology. Indeed it could be said that comparative ethology, at least when it addresses itself to questions about the evolutionary history of behaviour, applies the concepts and methods of comparative morphology to behaviour. However it is less easy to give a definition of behavioural homology than it is to give a definition of structural homology. A behavioural counterpart of the anatomical Principle of Connections would imply that items of behaviour regarded as homologous occupy the same positions in behaviour sequences sharing the same temporal organization or contextual relationships. Sequence and context have been utilized in judgments about behavioural homology, but they provide neither necessary nor sufficient criteria for such judgments. It has become apparent that evolution can change both the sequential position and context of occurrence of a behaviour pattern. Similarity of form of motor patterns has been the most frequently adduced support for claims of behavioural homology, but this too is inadequate as a defining criterion. There has apparently been both divergence and convergence in behavioural evolution, as there has in anatomical evolution, so that there are instances of behaviour patterns regarded as homologous that do not look very much alike, and instances of behaviour patterns that are similar but are not regarded as homologous. Similarity of form is usually backed up, at least implicitly, by independent evidence of common origin, such as the morphological evidence that has been used in arriving at conclusions about phylogenetic relationships between different kinds of animals. For example, in all species of gull that have been studied, turning of the head to face away from the other bird is a species-typical component of agonistic and courtship behaviour (Figure 1). Such a movement also occurs in similar contexts in the Common Crane and in some species of duck. The facing-away displays of the different species of gull are regarded as homologous to one another but not to those of cranes or ducks, since the latter are phylogenetically remote from gulls.

Judgments about behavioural homology thus involve several different kinds of evidence, and the directions of inference vary from one case to another. Arguments about common origins and even taxonomic affinity have been based on comparisons of the forms of behaviour; interpretations of similarities and differences of form and contextual occurrence of behaviour patterns have been influenced by accepted views about taxonomic affinity.

The possibility of circular argument is obvious, and it must be admitted that the concept of behavioural homology is less rigorous or precise than one is accustomed to demand in science. It is a rather vague concept. Nevertheless its use has led to plausible accounts of behavioural evolution, and it is difficult to see how such accounts could have been forthcoming without some notion of behavioural homology. Behavioural homology is a concept that still has 'open texture'; it is better represented by its *'logic in use'* (Kaplan, 1964) than by an attempt at complete and explicit definition.

The application of the comparative approach to the evolutionary history of behaviour is perhaps best illustrated by studies of 'ritualization.' Ritualization is the evolutionary modification of behaviour in the service of a signal function. By comparison of behaviour patterns in distantly and closely related species, and comparison of behaviour in different contexts within the range of behaviour shown by a single species, Lorenz, Tinbergen, and others arrived at the conclusion that display behaviour can be interpreted as 'derived activity' (Tinbergen, 1952).

For example, a display posture called the 'upright' has been observed and described in all species of gull that have been studied except the Kittiwake. A gull in this posture stands with its neck stretched vertically upwards, its bill horizontal or pointed slightly up or down, the carpal joints of its wings held away from the sides of the body, and its plumage 'sleeked' (Figure 2). The display occurs in agonistic and courtship contexts. The actions most often preceding and following its occurrence are attacking and fleeing. Its function is threat, except in courtship contexts in which this meaning appears to be qualified by subtle accompaniments in such a way that it promotes pair formation. The similarities in form, sequential position, context of occurrence and function of the uprights of different species, and the fact that they constitute one of a set of display types shared by the different species, have been adduced as evidence that they are homologous and hence have a common evolutionary origin. Analysis of the form of the posture has led to the interpretation that it consists of a mixture of 'frozen' components of attack behaviour: the lifted head corresponds to the first part of the action of pecking down at an opponent, and the lifted carpals correspond to the first part of the action of wing-beating at the opponent. The sleeked plumage, on the other hand, is a sign of fleeing tendency. These correspondences between details of the display and components of the behaviour that tends to precede and follow its occurrence have suggested that the display '... must have originated as a mosaic of intention movements of attack, inhibited by escape tendencies' (Tinbergen, 1959). Further comparisons added support to this interpretation. The Kittiwake, which lacks an upright, has no downward pecking in its attack behaviour. The Great Skua has a version of the upright

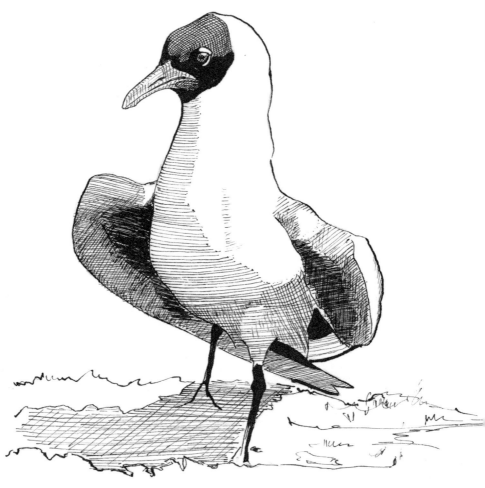

FIGURE 2 Upright display posture of a Black-headed Gull. (Drawn from a photograph)

which lacks lifting of the carpals, and this fits with the fact that it does not use wing-beating in fighting.

'Intention movements' – the initial parts of an action performed without leading into completion of the action – appear to have been one of the major evolutionary sources of displays. According to Daanje (1950) ritualization of the intention movements of taking off to fly has given rise to many of the social displays of birds. Tail-flicking in songbirds provides numerous examples of such displays (Andrew, 1956).

'Displacement activities' have apparently been another major source of displays. Displacement activities are activities that occur in contexts in which they do not seem to be functionally relevant and do not perform the function they ordinarily serve, e.g., grooming or nest-building movements occurring during fighting or courtship. There is debate about the causal basis of displacement activities, and it may well be that displacement activities constitute a causally heterogeneous category of behaviour. Be that as it may, there are numerous examples of display that show formal resemblances to grooming movements, nest-building movements, and so forth, and which occur in the kinds of conflict situations in which such movements occur as displacement activities. For example the threat display of the Three-spined Stickleback is little different from a nest-digging movement performed as a displacement activity and the obvious conclusion has been drawn that the display has been derived from the displacement activity (Tinbergen, 1951). Comparison of such behaviour in related species has, in some cases, suggested the evolutionary origin of a display which, taken by itself, defied interpretation. For example, in the Manchurian Crane the form of the threat display would not suggest that it is a ritualized preening movement, yet when it was compared with the threat displays of other species of crane it was seen to be homologous with patterns that link it, via a more or less continuous series of variations, to unritualized displacement preening (Lorenz, 1935). Lorenz interpreted this evidence as indicative of the course that evolution has taken in working on a displacement activity to change it into a form that serves the function of signalling threat.

Comparisons of display behaviour with what are believed to be its unritualized precursors have revealed that ritualization effects the kinds of changes that might be expected given the requirements for efficient signalling: salience and lack of ambiguity. Displays are typically conspicuous and stereotyped compared to their unritualized homologues. Conspicuousness and distinctiveness have been achieved by such changes as exaggeration of some components of movement with respect to others, increase or decrease in speed of performance, rhythmic repetition, and loss of some components. There may also be the addition of 'morphological support' such as brightly coloured or contrasting patches of plumage, crests, plumes, or frills. Stereotyping of motor patterns has apparently been assisted by elimination of their variation in response to the variation which occurs in the strength of eliciting factors – that is, the evolution of 'typical intensity' (Morris, 1959). Selection, presumably against inter-species hybridization, has tended to favour inter-species distinctness in homologous reproductive displays. Lorenz (1951) has shown that the pair-formation behaviour of ducks consists of a set of displays, present in more or less complete form in each species, but the homologous displays differ in details of form, timing, morphological support, and sequential position.

Whether the interpretations of comparative behavioural evidence referred to here are found acceptable will depend upon both their plausibility and the credulity of the reader. Where alternative interpretations suggest themselves it is not possible to decide the issue by experiment. The evolutionary interpretations to be put upon comparisons of behaviour patterns, even of closely related species, are often far from obvious and may be subject to controversy. The kinds of difficulties encountered are illustrated by a study of Blest (1957) in which detailed comparisons were made of the anti-predator wing-flashing displays of moths. Blest distinguished a variety of patterns but found that the distribution of the different types among the various species did not conform in any obvious systematic way to the accepted taxonomic affinities of the species. On the one hand some taxonomically closely related species showed quite different types of display patterns; on the other hand similar or virtually identical display patterns were found in distantly related species. So Blest had to draw the conclusion that there has been a remarkable degree of divergence and convergence within these insects in the evolution of the protective displays. Evolutionary interpretation of the evidence was consequently difficult and complicated. Nevertheless Blest was able to make a plausible case for the thesis that the displays originated from intention movements of flight, and he drew up a genealogy of their evolutionary succession.

This example, however, made Blest hesitant about the value of evolutionary interpretations of behaviour. Of necessity, arguments which use the concepts of behavioural homology and ritualization are indirect, since only the end products of behavioural evolution are ever available for observation. Exceptions to this are found in one or two rather special circumstances, such as in the preservation of behaviour effects in the form of nest structures when compared with, for example, fossil termite nests (Schmidt, 1958). In a review of the topic of ritualization Blest (1961, 103) went so far as to say that since '... there is no fossil record of micro-evolutionary changes in behaviour ... any statement about specific evolutionary events in a given group ... is never likely to be more than an inspired guess.' However the pattern of arguments about behavioural evolution would not be essentially different if there were a fossil record of behaviour. As in comparative morphology, so in comparative ethology, evolutionary interpretations of the facts are 'best fit' kinds of arguments. Their plausibility depends upon the success with which they fit the facts together economically and stand up to scrutiny for logical consistency. If the evolutionary history of behaviour is to be admitted as a viable subject of study at all, it is difficult to see what alternative there is to the comparative approach of ethology.

Most of my comments to this point have been concerned with the evolution of behaviour at the lowest taxonomic levels — species, genera, and so forth. It is only at these micro-evolutionary levels that the concept of behavioural homology, vague as it is, can be used with any degree of confidence. As one moves to comparisons at higher taxonomic levels the concept becomes progressively restricted in its applicability, and in comparisons between phyla it is of virtually no use at all.

This point has implications for the attempt to arrive at ideas about the evolution of human behaviour on the basis of comparison with other species, particularly if those species are as far away from man as insects, fish, or birds. Konrad Lorenz has made some of the most sophisticated analyses of evolution of behaviour at micro-evolutionary levels. He has also based ideas about human development, human motivation and the evolution of human behaviour on studies of geese, fish, and so forth, employing essentially the same kinds of argument as in the micro-evolutionary studies, but employing them in a context where the comparative concepts cannot be applied (Lorenz, 1966). Instead of argument by homology we end up with argument by vague analogy. The farther one goes from micro-evolutionary levels in attempting to arrive at ideas about the evolutionary history of behaviour, the more uncertain the grounds for evolutionary speculation become and the more warily one must proceed, because the guidance of the ancient comparative concepts is no longer available.

ERNST W. HANSEN

10 Some Aspects of Behavioural Development in Evolutionary Perspective*

Considerations of group structure in primates usually focus on the general properties of the group and deal with factors such as sex ratios, dominance hierarchies, the role the individual plays in the group, and the feeding and movement patterns of the group. The adaptive significance of such factors and evolutionary considerations of the general structure of naturally-evolved groups depend primarily upon data gathered in the field to reflect adequately environmental influences (e.g., Crook and Gartlan, 1966; Crook, 1970). The laboratory study of primate behaviour however, has the advantage of permitting the investigator to study more readily the development of behaviour in individual animals for prolonged periods of time. Studying the process of behavioural development itself may provide both insight into the operation of evolutionary forces and an understanding of group structure in the species concerned.

Clark (1959), in an over-all view of the primate order, has stated that the existing primates can be placed in a linear series which approximates the evolutionary history of the order. When this is done, one of the trends in primate evolution that emerges when 'lower' and 'higher' primates are compared is a retardation of the rate of development (see Schultz, 1965). The term *neoteny* or *foetalization* (deBeer, 1940) has been used to describe such a trend when there is a retardation of the rate of development of body structures relative to the rate of development of reproductive system. Mason (1968) has shown effectively how this concept can apply to behavioural development and he has shown that it is very closely associated with the increasing complexity seen in the behavioural development of higher primates. In particular, the same author has presented evidence that the self-directed stereotypic behaviour patterns seen in the rhesus monkey, the chimpanzee, and the human, because of differential rates and complexities of behavioural development, belie the phylogenetic standing of the individual exhibiting the

* Contribution number 111 from the Institute of Animal Behavior. The author's research program is supported by a grant (MH-17052) from the National Institute of Mental Health

behaviour. That is, the stereotyped behaviours of the rhesus monkey are less complex and varied and subject to less variability in their development than are the corresponding patterns of the chimpanzee. Similarly, the stereotyped behaviours of the chimpanzee are less complex and varied than are those of the human.

It is reasonable to argue that the retardation of the rate of behavioural development in primates is linked with, and perhaps ultimately causally related to, aspects of the learning that is necessary to ensure the 'proper' development of the individual, and the integration of the individual into the social group. During the increasingly prolonged period of development that we see in higher primates, the individual actively explores both the social and non-social aspects of his environment, and develops the behaviour patterns necessary for effective interaction with that environment.

Now, anyone who has watched monkey development will attest to the fact that a considerable amount of time is devoted to playful activities. Play, however, is not an easily defined item of behaviour despite the fact that it is an item about which monkey observers can reach some agreement. Two observers can sit and watch a group of monkeys and agree that the animals are playing rather than doing something else. One important aspect or characteristic of play is that we tend to think of it as being particularly associated with young animals and we are less disposed to think of play in adult interactions. Eibel-Eibesfeldt (1970), in placing play in broad comparative perspective, regards play as a special type of behaviour appearing almost exclusively in higher mammals and some birds. One could argue the question, but more facts and greater precision in terminology are needed. Within mammals, and especially primates, one could contend that corresponding to an increased period of dependency, increased emphasis is placed upon play activities. However, the investigations that have been done on play activities in primates seem barely to have scratched the surface with respect to the potential knowledge that is available concerning the particulars of how play activity may involve the key to understanding behavioural development.

Harlow and his associates at Wisconsin, particularly in their earlier work (Harlow and Harlow, 1965, 1968) have shown the over-all importance of play activity by manipulating peer experience. They have shown that, in an over-all sense, adequate peer group experience which includes play is essential to normal development. In addition, Dr Harlow indicates elsewhere in this volume that play is now even being used therapeutically. Thus, we have another general indication of the over-all importance of play, but lack a consideration of some of the specifics of how this activity can have the impact on development that it apparently does. What do we really know about the activities which we classify as play and why do we know so little?

Part of the problem underlying the answers to these questions appears to be that the motivational basis for play is an enigma. Why should animals want to play? This paper does not really propose to provide an adequate answer to this question, but it should be pointed out that a proper and complete answer would be of enormous significance to the understanding of behavioural development. These remarks are addressed to some of the things that are at least relevant to an answer to this question, when it is viewed in evolutionary perspective.

Hamburg (1962, 1968), in dealing with a discussion of the evolution of emotion, cited the example of an infant monkey clinging to his mother. He made the point of his articles in a variety of ways, but most emphatically by saying that the monkey 'wants to do what in fact he has had to do, over the course of many generations.' The point here is both simple and basic, and to mimic Hamburg's argument one could say that if it is important for the animal to play, the animal must want to play. It seems short-sighted to attempt to consider the evolution of behaviour without at least a corresponding consideration of the evolutionary basis of the motivation underlying such behaviour patterns. Looking at behaviour patterns, we all too often ignore the underlying motivational or emotional elements which, like anatomical structures or the behavioural patterns themselves, are subject to evolutionary pressures.

As an example, if we compare the structure of the hand of the rhesus monkey and the chimpanzee, the hand of the rhesus monkey is structurally better equipped to manipulate objects than is the hand of the chimpanzee. The apes, including the chimpanzee, have undergone a specialization associated with brachiation and semi-brachiation, so that the structure of the chimp's hand is not as well suited for opposition of digits essential for effective manipulation, as is the hand of the rhesus monkey. However, if we look at the behaviour of the chimpanzee and of the rhesus monkey, we see that the chimpanzee is, in fact, a better manipulator. How can this be explained — other than by saying the chimpanzee is more intelligent, or more curious, or has underlying capacities which far exceed the rhesus monkey's, which enable him to compensate for his structural handicap? The underlying basis for the behaviour outweighs the anatomical consideration. If, in the case of play behaviour, it is important for the species to play, the motivation underlying such behaviour must be as important as — if, perhaps, not more important than — the motor patterns themselves.

One could well ask: Why is it important for the species that individual monkeys develop play behaviour? Having already alluded to a supposed relationship between play (or peer experience) and social adjustment, the following may shed some light on this. Play, for the developing individual, serves both the purpose of getting the animal to know members of his social group, and to know himself. The non-serious nature of play seems to be the ideal format for the development of such knowledge. Although the motor activities appearing in the context of social play of the rhesus monkey appear themselves to be at least as complex as any other behaviour patterns seen in this species, it is within this context that much more than a series of motor patterns first appears and subsequently develops. Play also provides a format for social interaction which requires the animal to repeatedly and irregularly modulate his activities, especially in accordance with the behaviours exhibited by another individual. Frequently, play involves rapid tempo changes. The motor patterns involved may be secondary to the emotional or the motivational orchestration that occurs.

In short, play must indeed be serious non-seriousness — or it could not serve its function. The individual must learn the interrelationships between his internal, motivational, emotional, and arousal states, and his behaviour. He also has to learn how these internal states can be incorporated into interaction with another individual who is undergoing a similar development.

The consequences of this complex development within the individual contributes considerably to what we see as a high degree of individualization in the primates we work with. The primates, especially higher primates, have a large number of degrees of freedom in the developmental process, and the end product of the way a particular animal puts it all together, so to speak, provides for the great individual differences that we see in our subjects. Indeed, the existence of individual differences in primates, which to many are a hindrance to research on primates, are very much the outcome of evolutionary process acting on behavioural development. Rather than noise in a system that we wish to study, individual variation may be *the* aspect of primate interactions that should be of major concern to us.

My own experience with rhesus monkeys has led me to come to regard each animal as a distinct individual. I can readily think of the 'personality' of each animal I work with. Furthermore, I have developmentally studied a number of groups, and each group has its own idiosyncratic properties. If I were to be given data summaries describing the groups without naming the individuals involved, it would be possible to indicate without any difficulty which group and which individuals the summary concerned on the basis of behaviours that were exhibited. This reflects once more the individuality and nature of the specific individual relationships which are established within a group.

In addition, it could be suggested that the establishment of specific individual relationships leads to increasing complexity of social interactions which, because of these relationships, take on new dimensions. The animals thereby readily develop interactive patterns in which the relationship between two animals is very much influenced by not only the 'personalities' of each of them, but also the presence or attention, of one or more other animals. Moreover, it is not just another animal that is there, it is a specific individual that is there. The relations of each of the first two animals to the rest of the animals are important in influencing the entire interaction. A consideration of the nature of the complexity of such influences in primate interactions represents the key to an understanding of the higher order social structuring that we see in primate groups.

Many of the above factors — social learning, motor and motivational development, and individualization — are very closely linked. They are also the product of the retardation of the rate of behavioural development. It must, however, be emphasized that the contention that the behavioural-motivational co-ordination that appears in play can be and has been subject to selective pressure and has led to social groups whose nature is very much determined by the individual characteristics of their members.

One could not try to claim exclusiveness for the relationship between play and individualization in behavioural development. It is probable, for example, that mother/infant relationships and the variability associated therewith contribute a good portion to the nature of individual development. It is also quite possible, however, that natural selection has acted upon mother/infant relationships to strengthen them to the point where variability is limited, and a corresponding situation has not occurred with respect to the individual interactions which you see in play activities. In other words, the processes of evolution might well put a ceiling on the variability in maternal care that one could obtain and still have a viable monkey to work with, whereas such constraints would not equally apply to play.

DANIEL S. LEHRMAN

11   Can Psychiatrists use Ethology?

The remarks in this paper go beyond micro-evolution and comparisons between closely related species, to consider some general problems involved in the use of animal data, of the kind that psychiatrists hear from ethologists, for illuminating the human condition.

A question could properly be raised about what an ethologist is. The root word 'ethology' itself has a rather chequered history. It used to have, like the word 'drive,' a very simple and clear meaning which anyone could have defined. The term came into general use in Europe during the 1930s as a reflection of the development of a set of ideas formulated by Konrad Lorenz (1970), and by Niko Tinbergen (1951), who began to work collaboratively with Lorenz in the mid 1930s. They were zoologists and developed a school of zoological workers concerned with animal behaviour which had active centres in several European countries (Germany, Holland, England) where a fairly unified set of ideas developed, around such terms as 'innate releasing mechanism' and 'fixed action pattern.' In the United States at that time work on the behaviour of animals was mostly associated with psychologists. Whether animal psychologists or comparative psychologists, they were mostly interested in using animals as tools or objects for the study of what they regarded as problems of general psychology. With respect to these problems a variety of animals could be used, resulting in people running rats in mazes, cats in problem boxes, and so on. The ethologists had a different orientation. They dealt with problems that were posed by the way in which the animal acted in its natural environment. There was not much real communication between these two groups, except to the extent that individual people kept themselves informed about what was going on on the other side of the ocean.

What has happened in the last twenty years is that there has developed such a spread and interpenetration of ideas between the two groups of people that the distinctions between psychologically-oriented and zoologically-oriented students of animal behaviour have become blurred, as each group has become more aware of the problems, formulations, and strategies of the other

(Hinde, 1970). We find that if we call together, for any purpose, a group of people that it would be appropriate to speak of as engaged in ethological research, we find some people whose background is entirely in zoology, some whose background is psychology, and some with a mixed background. To characterize what is an appropriate set of people to whom to apply the term 'ethologists' is not possible on the basis of academic discipline. To the degree that it can be done at all, it would be on the basis of a set of common attitudes orienting them toward the problems of studying animal behaviour.

In general, I would say that one would be justified in referring to a person as an ethologist if he were interested in the study of animal behaviour in such a way as to be aware, as a primary background for his work, of the total behaviour pattern of the animal in relation to its natural environment; if the form of the problems that he dealt with were in some way dictated by the behaviour of the animal in its natural environment and arose in some way from an appreciation of the fact that the behaviour of the animal, like its morphology and physiology, constitutes a part of the way it has adapted to its natural environment; if he were therefore aware of the fact that animals who live in different environments are likely to be different in their behaviour as they are likely to be different in their morphology; and if he had an appreciation of the fact that behaviour has evolved in the course of evolution, in the sense in which morphology has. There are all sorts of behaviour about whom some, but not all, of these things are true. One cannot be very specific about who is an ethologist and who is not. However, the people themselves do not have any great difficulty in deciding about the sorts of people with whom they want to communicate.

I have had many contacts with psychiatrists and psychotherapists over the last ten or fifteen years, since it became fashionable for psychiatrists to pay attention to the field of animal behaviour. I have continued to ask myself: What exactly is it that psychiatrists would like to have, that they would think helpful, from ethologists? It is not an easy question to answer. I can think of an analogous situation in some of my own reactions to fields of study other than my own. I am concerned with understanding the organization of behaviour in the animals with which I work, and I like to understand them in as much depth as I feel capable of achieving. This means not only watching behaviour and doing experiments with situations when it occurs, or about the effects of different kinds of experience on it, but thinking about the physiological mechanisms in the animal which account for the organization of the behaviour that is seen. Therefore, although my prime interest is in animal behaviour, I have to look a good deal in the neurophysiological and endocrinological literature.

Considering how I deal with the neurophysiological literature, it is rather amusing to think about how the psychiatrist conceives of the relevance of the field of animal behaviour. If the neurophysiologist is interested, for example, in the physiology of the visual system there will be a wide variety of kinds of neurophysiological evidence which will seem to him to bear upon how the visual system works. He will be interested in, and must know about, the details of the way in which the sensory elements in the retina are connected to each other and are, in turn, connected to elements slightly higher in the retina. He will have to know about the ways in which information and nerve impulses are transmitted from the eye to the brain. There will be a wide range of things with which he will become familiar: biochemical studies of light-induced transformations in retinal substances, the anatomy of synaptic connections, the organization of the visual system inferred from evoked potentials, and the influence of damage to different parts of the brain on a wide variety of visually affected responses. Although there will be many things about the nervous system which seem important to him, as a neuro-physiologist, in order to understand how the visual system works, he may not be interested in behaviour at all.

When I look at that literature, much of it seems to be boring and irrel-evant. My eye gets caught primarily by things that seem to have an iso-morphic relationship with things that concern me. For example, if a paper is addressed directly to the fact that a complex configuration of stimuli has a simple describable effect upon the activation of specific nerve cells in the central nervous system, it immediately strikes me as capable of throwing some light on the question of how a bird can be constructed so that it can respond selectively to one kind of head movement made by its young or its mate, but not to another. In this case, the neurophysiologist has presented evidence which seems to me like a possible neurophysiological explanation of something like stimulus-specificity in a complex social situation. However, I may be unaware of the connections which the neurophysiologist sees between that mechanism and nervous system events which are not obviously related to behaviour, and which do not therefore attract my attention, even though they may have an immediately perceivable relationship to the neuro-mechanisms of the visual system and thus do attract the attention of a neuro-physiologist interested in visual physiology. I may then be picking out from the whole body of neurophysiological work a piece of evidence which becomes encapsulated in my mind as a neurophysiological explanation of a behavioural phenomenon in which I am interested. This is valid to the extent that the evidence is relevant to the phenomenon, but, unaware of relation-ships appreciated by the neurophysiologist and of no interest to me because they are not behavioural, I may misinterpret it in a way which distorts its essence as seen by people who work with it as a professional object. This is a danger, particularly in the biological sciences, whenever any scientist deals with the work of professionals in another area which has glancing, spotty, or localized relevance to his problems.

The best protection against that kind of distortion is, of course, for the student of behaviour to become as familiar with the physiology of the nervous system as the neurophysiologist is. This is not possible, so there is no perfect protection. Attempts to provide it to some degree involve reading widely in the literature, broadening one's perception of relationships on slightly different levels, and thus increasing the range of things that can be appreciated independently of their direct relevance to one's own research interest. There is no end to what one must learn about all fields of science for protection against the misinterpretation of neurophysiological, biochemical, endocrinological, neuroendocrinological, anatomical, ecological, and evolutionary evidence. They all bear on the study of behaviour. One must be selective, but any selectivity reimposes the original danger.

Another solution is to have enough association with professionals who are neurophysiologists, biochemists, or students of evolution that you frequently talk about the sorts of things you each do. This is difficult, because we tend to develop our most intimate professional relationships with people who are interested in problems at a level that we think is most interesting and most important. It seems that there are only imperfect and partial ways of guarding against the distortions involved in using professional information from one level to elucidate problems at another. This is a problem which is, as I am being eleborately careful to point out, not restricted to psychiatrists trying to interpret for their own use the results of animal behaviour studies.

As an example, we are commonly asked how animal data can be used to understand aggression. The way in which the sources of aggression in human beings are not only transformed, but arise in the course of social experience, does not leave us with any great hope that simple formulations about the way in which an animal has its hostility turned on and off by signals from other animals (in the way that we describe the behaviour of gulls) really would be very useful in dealing with human behaviour. It is sometimes difficult to understand why psychoanalysts who come into intimate contact with the sources of complex human interactions in their practice feel that the experience of people who work with animals is likely to provide a more valid guide to what is happening with their patients than their own experience.

What does it mean to interpret the behaviour of one kind of animal by reference to the behaviour of another kind of animal? Can we make interpretations by looking at 'equivalent' processes? Can we appropriately and meaningfully look at an event or partial organization in one animal species (e.g., the rhesus monkey) and use that to increase our understanding of an 'equivalent' or, for us, a phenomenonally identical process in another animal such as (to take another example at random) the human?

This question may be approached by digressing to a very different species. The case involves a simple and familiar animal, the American cowbird, a common blackbird. There are many species of blackbird in North America. We could ask the question: How does a blackbird get to know what kind of bird it ought to mate with? It moves around and sees different kinds of birds; it meets blackbirds of its own species; it meets blackbirds of other species; it meets sparrows, both white-crowned and song sparrows; it meets warblers, vireos, and thrushes; and the question is: How does it get to choose a mate which is a blackbird of its own species?

Natural selection is going to be working very hard indeed to make sure that the bird does not mate with a member of any other species, because mating between members of different species is liable to lead to offspring which are adapted neither to the environment of the mother species nor to the environment of the father species, and will therefore not survive as well anywhere as either of the parents. That is a simple statement of a rather complex situation which is involved in the very biological definition of the species. We can assume that, in a normal environment, natural selection works to eliminate any genes which would have the result of allowing the animal to mate with members of other species. But how does this happen? We could ask the experimental question: Does an animal learn anything in its early life which helps it to mate with its own species?

It is probable that the redwinged black bird is influenced by its experience in selecting a mate. Older redwinged blackbirds who, presumably, have had more experience, are more selective in choosing to mate only with a dummy of a female redwinged blackbird rather than with any other kind of dummy, such as a male redwinged blackbird or a cowbird, than are younger animals.

Consider, however, the cowbird. The cowbird and the redwinged blackbird are closely related, being different genera in the same family. They are closely enough related that in learning to identify at sight the birds in the neighbour-hood, one of the things that would cause some difficulty would be confi-dently distinguishing between a female redwinged blackbird and a female cowbird, or even, for some between a male redwinged blackbird and a male cowbird. Yet if a cowbird is reared with birds of other species, it mates only with cowbirds.

These are two very closely related animals. One of them, the redwinged blackbird, learns from its parents and siblings something about with whom to mate when it grows up. It seems, however, that the cowbird does not. Were we to be asked the general question about whether early experience plays a role in determining species identification, intraspecies association, or mate selection in birds, we would reach entirely opposite conclusions from studies of the two species. What is the difference between them? The cowbird is a brood parasite, or social parasite, like the European cuckoo. The female cowbird, instead of building a nest, lays her eggs in the nest of a host bird of another species. Every cowbird in existence has been brought up by foster parents of another species. Every redwinged blackbird has been brought up by parents of its own species.

If there is a general tendency in the genus to which the redwinged black-bird belongs to learn things from early experience, and if the blackbird had its choice of mate determined in part by experience with parents and siblings during early life (experience, as pointed out by Marler, in this volume, con-strained by its perceptual organization and structure), then the redwinged blackbird would not mate very often with other than redwinged blackbirds because, if it mates with what it has associated with when young, it will mate with the redwinged blackbird. However, if a cowbird were in the least influ-enced in the choice of a mate by this kind of early experience it would tend to have offspring which could not survive because they were neither cow-birds, redwinged blackbirds, rusty blackbirds, nor melodious blackbirds.

In order for hybridization to be eliminated by natural selection, it is necessary that natural selection should eliminate any tendencies in the cow-bird to take advantage of its early experience in learning to mate. But this is not the case in the redwinged blackbird. These are two animals which have strikingly different processes in their development leading toward the selec-tion of a mate. There is clearly a difference in their relationships between the role of experience and that of nervous system maturation in determining this very important aspect of their respective behaviour patterns. Therefore, inter-preting the behaviour of one of these birds by reference to the behaviour of the other (not by interpreting the movement patterns they use in courting, but in determining the processes that lead to the selection of a mate) would lead to a serious error. If, rather than attending solely to the role of early experience in determining the selection of a mate and comparing the two animals in this respect, we tried to see first what mate selection in each one of those animals had to do with the total pattern making up its life; and if, instead of comparing the equivalent processes, details, or areas of behaviour in the two and thus incorrectly surmising what was going on in each, we were to compare the total *pattern* of the life of each animal, including the process in question; then each *pattern* would give us some perspective about the organization of, and about the ecological significance of, the other pattern, which would be more valuable than the perspective we could get about either by studying it alone.

One may ask what all this has to do with attachment behaviour in monkeys. Consider that a rhesus monkey is seriously disturbed by being separated from its mother and that this disturbance lasts for a long time (Spencer-Booth and Hinde, 1967). Then, consider that a human baby in London, or in Cambridge, Massachusetts, is seriously disturbed in ways which seem similar, by being separated from its mother (Bowlby, 1969). What is the appropriate way to link those two observations? It has been remarked by Charles Kaufman that in different species of macaque there are, in general, different tendencies for the animals to remain in contact with each other. These differences in tendency, regardless of their origin, are reflected in a striking species difference in the ease with which a baby monkey can make contact with an adult other than its mother. Consider the fact that when young bonnet macaques and pigtail macaques are removed from their mothers the pigtail young do not make contact with another adult, while the bonnet do. Consider that in the species in which the young *do* make contact with the adult, there appears to be an amelioration of the effects of separation even to the degree of leaving out the last severe stage of the withdrawal response. Dr Kaufman points out elsewhere in this volume that he plans to see whether these two species differ with respect to the long-term effects of separation upon emotionality and personality. In these closely-related species of macaque, there are quite different immediate as well as later effects of separation from the mother. We could not interpret those different effects without knowing about the differences in life patterns and in social relationships of these animals. How the species differ in the degree of physical contact which depends upon the early experience of the infant – that is, how it becomes a bonnet or a pigtail in this respect – is another question Dr Kaufman will be examining. We do not yet know the extent to which the experience of associating with parents in that kind of group enables an infant to make or avoid contact with members of the group.

In the human case, when a mother is withdrawn from an infant in a place like England or Cambridge, it occurs in a situation in which the extended family has all but disappeared. The character of the nuclear family is presumably affected. When the mother goes to hospital it does not seem self-evident that the father ought not to go to work, because the work is important and there are other people to take care of the child. Compare that situation with the Samoan culture, in which the family is so extended that there are very large numbers of people who seem, in rather important ways, to be equivalent parents to a child (Mead, 1928). Children move very readily from one set of adults to another, and the warmth of personal relationships spreads over a much wider area than in our culture with its particular kind of nuclear family. The separation data in a culture such as that would perhaps seem less striking than in our western culture.

The rhesus monkey, not for cultural, social or historical reasons but, at least in part, for genetical ones, differs from the bonnet monkey in ways which are reminiscent of, and seem relevant to, the ways in which the Samoan and British cultures differ, not for biological reasons but for cultural and historical ones. In this light, the separation data for the rhesus monkey and what we have been pleased to call the human case take on a different perspective in each instance than they would when interpreted in the context of the immediately surrounding pattern alone. If we keep in mind simultaneously the differences among the different monkey species, the differences among human cultures, and the similarity between the rhesus monkey data and the Western European/North American data, it is possible to see in perspective an important fact: that separation from a parent-figure is extremely distressing, and has important after-effects, in the absence of a social setting that makes amelioration possible.

There *is* something, however, which this perspective may prevent. That is the conclusion that, because separation from the mother is traumatic to the child, the mother is obligated to spend all of her time taking care of the child *for reasons arising from the biological nature of the human species.* Had Harry Harlow worked on the bonnet monkey, and Robert Hinde been attracted to it because of information provided by Harlow about its care and because interesting results emerge from such studies of early infant experience, we might have a somewhat different conception about what biology says on the appropriate roles for women. Concluding from these data that biology tells us we are violating our inherent nature, in ways which are bound to be discordant, if the woman does not spend all her time caring for the baby while the man does important things like programming computers; and concluding that it is our biological nature that demands this kind of sex role differentiation — that it is a violation of natural selection and of Darwin's theories for a woman to feel as seriously about her work as a man — may be using what look like scientific considerations simply to justify our social prejudices.

I have been asked whether there is any evidence among animals of rejection or resentment about being restricted to the maternal role. Answering in the negative, I have wondered, 'What does it mean to say that I do not know of any such evidence?' The questioner usually implies that the development of such a resistance, when it occurs in humans, is somehow an unbiological phenomenon — an abnormality. But all of us live in an unbiological, abnormal situation, if by normal we understand the primeval situation in the most remote sources of our evolutionary history. Consider the feelings recorded recently by a striking auto worker. He resented having his time governed by the rate at which the cars were going past him on the assembly line. That rate was somehow determined in such a way that when he became comfortable with it the line speed increased, because if he were comfortable with it that meant that he could do better. He expressed an intense resentment about the work that he has to do in order to provide food for his children. Would one ask: 'Is there any evidence, among infrahuman animals, of males resenting the necessity to gather food and bring it back to the female and the young?' It would be inappropriate to ask, because the resentment at issue arises out of social relationships which have historical, and not biological origins. It would be unthinkable to reduce this to a question of whether the man accepted his male role and was therefore willing to live as a biological male. Perhaps the question of willing acceptance of the solely nurturing female role is not of exactly that order and the absurdity of asking such a question in the case of the female role has a different basis. Nonetheless, consider the way of life, for a woman and for a man, in our very highly evolved, technologically sophisticated, socially complicated, historically long-emerging culture. To say that the role of one person (the woman) in such a social situation is biologically determined, while the role of another person (the man) is socially determined, is asymmetrically simplifying the question. If animals do not show this resentment, I would infer that it is because there has been no evolution of a social situation in which there is any reason for it to develop in a large number of individuals, not that it is somehow abnormal when it does develop in a different social situation.

Irven DeVore has commented that male anthropologists are practically unaware of the little wooden stick with which the woman gathers eighty per cent of the food. I am aware that the discussion about Samoan culture, to which I referred, was produced by a woman anthropologist. Some might suggest that she may speak from a special woman's point of view so this sort of discussion must be regarded with some care. However, I wonder how many men who would say this recognize that what they say is also said from a point of view which does not seem special only because it has been massively authoritative, universal, and taken for granted. As DeVore has also said, these are things men do not like to talk about – and do not like to think about spontaneously. They do not think about matters of this kind unless women get very indignant about them, as is now sometimes the case. Similarly there are many things that some races of people know but do not really think about until other races become unpleasant about them.

The scientific aspect of this has to do with the question of whether interpretations across very different levels are best carried out by looking for part-processes which seem the same, so that, for example, by studying the attachment process at one level light can be thrown on how it works at another level, or whether interpretations must involve a wider appreciation of patterns. It is like asking: 'Can a psychiatrist really make optimum use of animal behaviour studies by paying attention to ethology in the way that I used to pay attention to neurophysiology, before I forced myself to pay a deeper kind of attention to it?' Would they, on the other hand, be making better use of ethology if they had a more continuous attention to the field, and a more continuous association with an ethologist, than is provided through the work of ethologists who think they should study mainly those items which will seem relevant to the psychiatrists? For example, an ethologist selecting data to present to psychiatrists, looking for the type and organization of data which would be most relevant and most interesting to them, may narrow down his focus from the ethology and ecology of a monkey group to something which would seem sufficiently similar to a human group situation that he appears justified in studying it.

A final statement of caution: to assume that animal work really can demonstrate the biologically appropriate differences between men and women is hazardous. It is, at best, naive to think that the fact that a father monkey spends his time protecting the troop while the mother takes care of the baby suggests that it is somehow inappropriate for a man to take time off from programming computers or talking to psychiatrists to make possible a widening of roles for the female of his species in a way which is technologically feasible. The human male's involvement in organizing universities, building industries, and making submarines is an enormously unbiological distortion of the original and immediately-perceptible relationship between the food-getting activity and getting of food. When men who do these things imply that God really intended women to stay home and take care of the babies, they remind me of the little old lady in a New Yorker cartoon who is offered a drink by an airline stewardess, and who says, 'No thank you. I do not believe God intended us to drink while flying.'

HARRY F. HARLOW

12 Induction and Alleviation of Depressive States in Monkeys

During the last two years we have initiated a research programme designed to induce or simulate various forms of human depression in rhesus monkeys. If monkeys can be made depressed for a prolonged period of time a variety of biological and social studies becomes possible. Prior to this particular programme, we had already conducted two studies on infantile or anaclitic depression produced by separating infant monkeys from their mothers at six months of age (Seay, Hansen and Harlow, 1962). This research had served as a model for other investigators testing the effects of infant separation from the mother and mother separation from the infant on rhesus, bonnet, and pigtail macaques.

SEPARATION: MOTHER IN SIGHT

In our original researches we separated pairs of infant friends from their respective mothers while the infant friends were playing together in a spacious play compartment (Figure 1). The mothers, meanwhile, were continuously confined to two living cages contiguous to the play area, the entrance to which was too small for the mothers to use. Mother/infant separation was achieved by inserting plexiglass slides between each of the two living cages and the play compartment when the infants had left their homes to play together. Thus, in this situation the mothers and infants were physically but not visually separated.

Both the separated infants and mothers were disturbed by these procedures, even though the intensity and duration of the disturbance was greater for the infants than for the mothers. Indeed, the infants' successive behaviours were startlingly reminiscent of the separation stages of protest and despair, as described by Bowlby (1960), following human mother/infant separation. Protest by the monkeys consisted of violent crying vocalizations, compulsive random locomotion, and assault directed against the offending plexiglas slide. After a day or so the frequency of the protest behaviours declined and behaviour patterns obviously portraying despair developed. These included a general decrease in activity and an increase in self-clasp and huddling behaviours.

Objective time-sampling records were continued for three-week periods before, during, and after separation. These data revealed that play activities were almost obliterated during the entire separation interval, even though they had been high before separation was begun, and again became frequent and intense shortly after separation ended (Figure 2). We believe that the inhibition of play was our most valid and meaningful measure of depression, and the differences in amount of play during separation contrasted to the amount of play both before and after separation were highly significant statistically.

SEPARATION: MOTHER OUT OF SIGHT

We conducted a second experiment which was essentially a replication of the first except for the fact that opaque fibreboard screens were substituted for the transparent plexiglas dividers placed between the two home cages and the play area. Here again the infants passed through Bowlby's stages of protest and despair, and play behaviour was significantly depressed during the separation period. However, much to our surprise, the intensity and probably the duration of the depression, as measured by the objective tests, was lower when sight of the mothers was entirely shut off from the infants' view, than when the plexiglass screens were used. It was as if the monkeys had heard of the notion 'out of sight, out of mind.'

SEPARATION: BETWEEN INFANTS

The breaking of any affectional bond should cause a strong separation reaction, and we had previously demonstrated that affection between mother and child was probably no stronger than affection among infant playmates. Working on this assumption, a Wisconsin graduate student, Mr Stephen Suomi, separated groups of four infants from each other, not once but for twelve consecutive sessions. The infants were together for three days per week and separated for four. Each separation of each infant group elicited violent protest responses of vocalization and increased movement, which were followed in about twenty-four hours by responses of despair, as indicated by self-clasp and huddle. Upon reunion the infants clasped each other tightly (Figure 3). Furthermore, there was no indication of adaptation to any of these stages of protest, despair, and reunion throughout the twelve sessions.

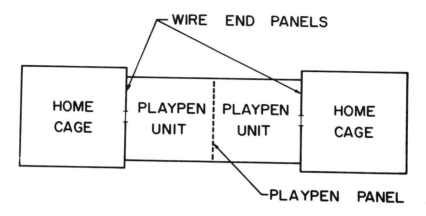

FIGURE 1   Deprivation apparatus

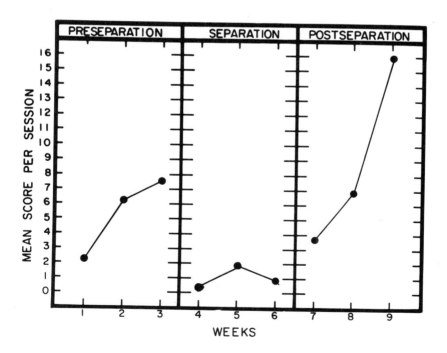

FIGURE 2   Infant approach-withdrawal play responses

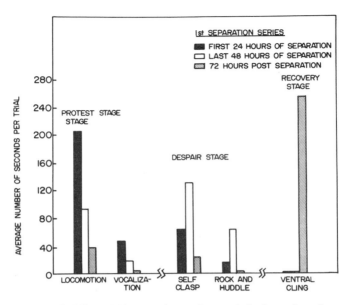

FIGURE 3 Effect of 12 separation sessions on behaviour of monkeys

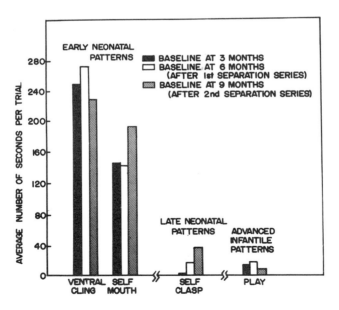

FIGURE 4 Arrest of behavioural maturation by repetitive separations

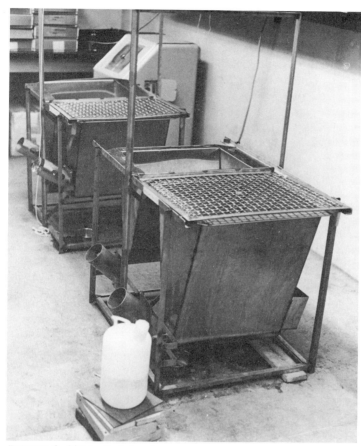

FIGURE 5   The vertical chamber

The reaction to the twelfth separation was no more or no less severe than to the first separation.

The behaviour of the separated infants when together was measured at three months of age, when separation began, and also at six and nine months of age, when the repetitive sessions were being conducted. Ventral clinging and self-mouthing, which are normal infantile behaviours at three months of age, showed no decrease in frequency at six months or nine months of age, when they should have been essentially non-existent. Contrary results were obtained for play, which is a behaviour that is just developing in normal monkeys at three months of age, but which attains high levels at six months and very high levels at nine months of age. In the repetitively separated monkeys the fragmentary play observed at three months failed to increase materially at six or nine months, an unheard-of-event for normal monkeys. These measures and other related measures show that twelve repetitive separations had stopped normal behavioural maturation and left the six- and nine-month-old monkeys in a state of infantilization or maturational arrest (Figure 4).

THE VERTICAL CHAMBER

In an effort to produce depression or depressive-like states by means other than repetitive separation, which is a relatively slow and time-consuming process, we created a special apparatus called the vertical chamber, a sloping vertical cage with a fine mesh bottom and a hardware cloth top (Figure 5). A group of monkeys, ranging from six to thirteen months of age, were individually confined in these chambers for a month, and their behaviours were measured for two subsequent months. Infantile behaviours of huddling and self-clasp remained high throughout this period, whereas more complex behaviours of locomotion and environmental exploration were greatly depressed (Figure 6). Thus depression was achieved with startling speed and was maintained for a significant time.

In the next study we compared the behaviour of monkeys that were confined to the vertical chamber for six weeks antecedent to ninety days of age with the behaviour of monkeys from two control groups, one raised in bare wire cages, and one raised with normal infant playmates. Again, the monkeys placed in the vertical chambers subsequently exhibited a high incidence of infantile behaviours of cling and huddle, behaviours which were almost non-existent in the other two groups (Figure 7). Contrariwise, complex behaviours of exploration, social contact, and play did not develop in the monkeys after release from the vertical chambers but developed normally in the members of the other two groups. The behaviour of these three groups of monkeys has now been traced for a year after release from the vertical chambers, and the long-term effects are clear. The monkeys placed in the vertical chambers show a high incidence of self-mouth, self-huddle, and self-clasp behaviours, whereas social contacts and play are almost non-existent. Contrariwise, the members of both the control groups show little or no self-mouthing, self-huddling, and self-clasping, and exhibit a high level of social contacts and play behaviour.

DEPRESSION

These behaviours of the chambered infants as they approached behavioural maturity might be described as either depressed or infantilized. Depression, of

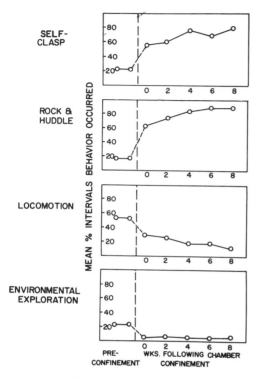

FIGURE 6   Effect of 30 days' pit experience on selected behaviours of four wire-cage-reared monkeys (age 6-13 mo.)

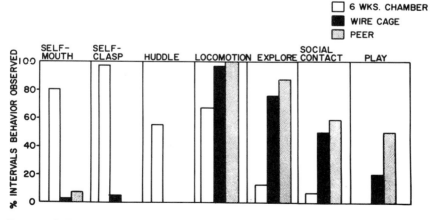

FIGURE 7   Playroom behaviours, 9-11 months of age

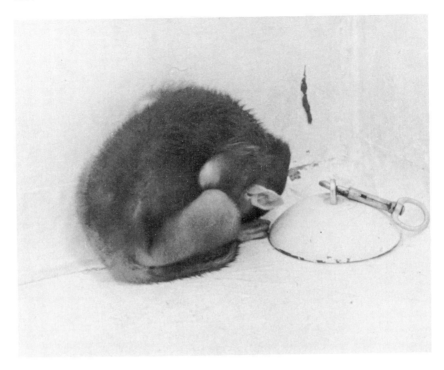

FIGURE 8   Depressed monkey infant

course, often involves regression or an exaggeration of infantile needs and behaviour, therefore, the two terms need not involve much controversy. By simply assuming that depression is a state of regression we might avoid controversy over terminology. Aside from terminology, it is obvious that a relatively brief state of semi-isolation in the vertical chamber produced abnormal behaviours that were remarkably stable in young monkeys (Figure 8).

THERAPY

Having demonstrated that depression or depressive-like abnormal states could be induced in monkeys by a number of means, we attempted to rehabilitate abnormal monkeys by the ministrations of other monkeys serving as 'therapists.'

Previous studies had demonstrated that monkeys raised from birth until six months of age in total isolation and then placed with age-mates were totally destroyed socially. The isolated monkeys avoided social contacts, they

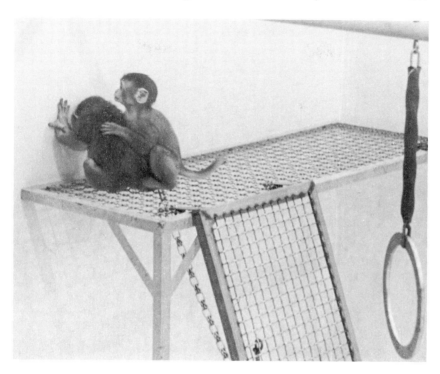

FIGURE 9   Isolate on left, therapist on right: Behaviour typical of early therapy session

did not play, and they were fearful and disturbed. Furthermore, these abnormal social behaviours persisted over periods of years and tended to
become exaggerated rather than improved with time. Sexual behaviour was
abnormal or non-existent and some reluctant females that were deviously
impregnated were inadequate or brutal mothers. The only vigorous trait that
developed was brief episodes of mixed fear with uncontrolled aggression
often directed toward infants. Aggression against infants is almost never seen
in normal adults. In this study we are assuming that six months' total isolation produced depression or a depressive state in monkeys.

When the social isolates were six months of age they were placed in quad
cages, which are large cages subdivided into four chambers and used for either
housing or social testing. The therapist monkeys had been raised in quad-cage
quadrants with a surrogate mother and had been allowed interaction with
age-mates during the first three months of life, a time at which play was
beginning to develop.

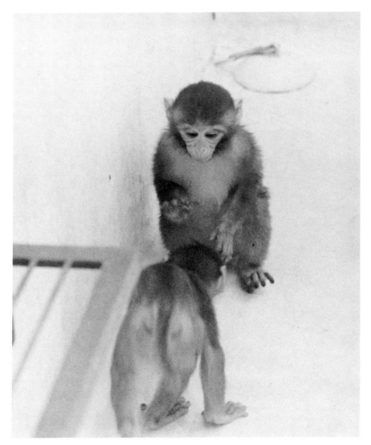

FIGURE 10   Therapy proceeds

Therapy sessions involved placing an isolated monkey with a younger therapist monkey twice a week in a quad cage, and twice a week in a large, unfamiliar playroom (Figure 9). Once a week two isolates and two therapists were placed in the playpen as a group of four.

RESULTS

The isolate monkeys rapidly overcame any fear that they originally had of the therapist monkeys and began to accept and even reciprocate body contact instead of withdrawing and huddling (Figure 10). Within a few weeks they

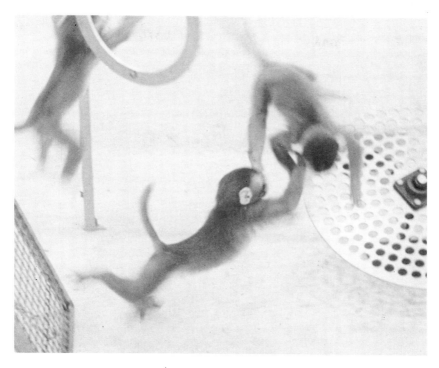

FIGURE 11   Isolate males engaging in rough-and-tumble play (a typical normal male monkey play pattern)

made little or no attempt to flee and began to reciprocate physical interaction. After six months of interaction, reciprocal play between isolates and therapists was not uncommon. Even after this time isolate animals occasionally showed abnormal posturing at the beginning or sometime throughout a test session.

By unavoidable accident both of the isolated monkeys were males and both of the therapist monkeys were females. Many years of testing monkeys in playrooms had taught us that the play patterns of male and female monkeys are fundamentally different. Male monkey play, in a pattern called rough-and-tumble play, involves a maximal amount of bodily contact, whereas female monkey play is characterized by chasing back and forth with bodily contact minimal or non-existent — a non-contact form of play. After the socially isolated monkeys and the therapists had come to live on equal terms as a group of four, we were astounded to realize that the isolate males played together and engaged in rough-and-tumble play (Figure 11), whereas the therapist females formed their own play group and engaged in non-contact play. The males could not have learned rough-and-tumble play from the females, who never played this way. By rehabilitating the males, the females had enabled the males to develop their own masculine heritage, which was above and beyond any simple act of female social imitation. These results, showing sex-characteristic differences in rhesus infant play behaviour, suggest that our interpretations follow the injunction: Render unto males the things that are males', and to females their foibles and fancies.

DAVID HAMBURG

13 Ethological Perspectives on Human Aggressive Behaviour[*]

There has been, of late, a great deal of interest in problems of aggression, much of it from an ethological point of view. Many readers of this publication will have read one or more of the recent books on the subject, and through them many have been stimulated to learn more about ethology. In the public at large, we see enormous concern about man's aggressive heritage, or about the corruption of his basically peaceful nature — updated versions of the old argument about whether man is fundamentally good or evil. Widely popular books by Lorenz (1966), Ardrey (1966), Morris (1967, 1969), and Storr (1968), and one edited by Ashley Montagu (1968) have entered into the lists of these controversies. While they are open to criticism, they do have some merit and serve to draw attention to an important area. Indeed, one can hardly imagine a problem more important than that of aggression. Moreover, these books have a welcome evolutionary orientation and there are some valuable items (such as John Crook's (1968) fine paper) embedded in them.

There are, however, serious disadvantages, some of which have been described by Robert Hinde. Some of these books scarcely utilize studies of man's closest living biological relatives — that is, the non-human primates — or, when they do, usually not the most recent studies. With few exceptions, there is no systematic or critical coverage of primate research in these volumes. Also (as Robert Hinde (1967) pointed out some time ago in a critique of Lorenz's book, *On Aggression*) most of them lack serious attention to developmental considerations. The use of human material is highly impressionistic, anecdotal, and inferential. There is little reliance on systematic human research, even where it exists in relative abundance. Despite these limitations, the social impact of such publications provides a fitting backdrop to the following remarks, which explore the subject of aggression somewhat further. Because views on it are readily associated with, and influenced by, strongly-held political convictions, aggression is very difficult to study

* This work was assisted by a grant from the Commonwealth Fund

objectively. The purpose of this paper is to call attention to a few promising lines of enquiry that link evolutionary and developmental considerations pertinent to human aggressiveness. This is an under-manned area of scientific work and any conclusions must be quite tentative.

THE ORIENTATION OF ETHOLOGY

To set this discussion in context, there are some aspects of the contribution of ethology to the study of human behaviour – particularly psychiatry – which deserve mention. These include, notably, its orientation and its methods. One of the important contributions of ethology has been to direct our attention to natural habitats. This has meant in ethology, in so far as possible, the habitat in which the organism has evolved. Another orientation of ethology that has been important is the relation of behaviour to ecological variability. It has been assumed and demonstrated that the same species does not behave in entirely the same way in different parts of its habitat. Similarly, the same group does not behave in the same way in the dry season as compared to the wet season, and so forth. Thirdly, there has been an emphasis on the evolutionary view of behaviour, particularly on behaviour as adaptation and, in this respect, a calling of attention to the group as well as the individual – that is, the ways in which the group meets the adaptive requirements of species survival.

In recent years we have come to pay more attention to adaptive tasks and strategies in studies of human behaviour. This may partially correct one of the mistakes made in western culture, which has been to take too much for granted that basic adaptive requirements would be readily met – food, sex, shelter, caring for young, and so on. In much of the world this cannot be taken for granted, and even in our own case there are important complexities there. An orientation to the adaptive tasks and strategies is helpful in understanding human behaviour. We must, of course, include considerations of self-esteem, and of significant inter-personal relationships, in this kind of approach.

THE INFLUENCE OF ETHOLOGY

These orientations of ethology have already had some impact and significant implications for those of us trying to move forward in understanding contemporary human behaviour. One has to do with the interview, the prime tool for psychiatrists and a major tool in other behaviour sciences. The interview provides us with a limited sample of behaviour. We are constantly trying to make some kind of transformation which would permit us to take account of the individual's behaviour in other settings as it appears to us through the interview. The notion of transference is one important such effort. In recent years, groups studying the families of schizophrenics have found it useful to provide other settings in which they could see these patients and significant others. They have not confined themselves to the traditional interview situation, but have devised special interviews and gone out to the home and to work situations. They have gone to different segments of the 'natural habitat' of contemporary man, where people live, where they spend much of their lives, where they invest their motivations and emotions, to see how behaviour looks in a variety of settings. To a certain extent that is an ethological influence – and a good one. Basically, this is direct observation in natural habitats.

Another major influence has been to view man as an organism. This has tended to break down the old, hoary, and not helpful barriers between biological and social science. More and more, under the influence of an ethological orientation, we see a meshing of biological and social considerations vis-à-vis contemporary man.

Thirdly, ethologists have been very clever about relatively simple experimental variations in the field. They have ventured into the natural habitat, tried to describe the behaviour carefully and systematically, and then varied certain elements that look significant, to see what the consequences will be. Students of human behaviour have a long way to go in this regard, but there are some ingenious things being attempted. For example, there are the experiments of Philip Zimbardo (1969) in New York City and Palo Alto. He reports that he left an old car with its hood up as a kind of distress signal, and its license plates off, on the street in two locations, middle-class neighbourhoods near Stanford and New York Universities, respectively. Observers then carefully recorded what happened to the car over the next three days – in effect, how rapidly it was destroyed. The findings (it was destroyed in New York and not damaged in Palo Alto) are themselves interesting, but what is equally important is the method – the originally ethological technique of getting out into the field and creating a simple variation in conditions. This may be a prototype for a sort of human ethology.

Finally, there are advantages in animal studies per se. As pointed out elsewhere in this volume by Dr Hinde, there are almost insurmountable ethical, financial, and technical difficulties about investigating, for example, the question of whether early mother/infant separation may permanently alter something in the brain or the endocrine system. In a number of important problems, the only rational approach would be to study animals, trying to include some that are closely biologically related to man, and then using the results of those studies as a guide to tell us where to look in man. Of course, ultimately, if we are interested in man we will have to answer these questions in human subjects. However, our justification − ethically, financially, and technically − is very much stronger if we go to man after we have learned where to look, so to speak, by studying closely-related species.

AGGRESSION IN PRIMATES

We have been especially interested in observation of baboon and chimpanzee patterns of threat and attack in natural habitats. The question has been: what are the conditions under which chimpanzees and baboons are most likely to threaten and attack other animals, primarily within their own species, but also in other species? Let us first consider the case of the chimpanzee. Goodall's (1968) observations are a unique resource in this field. The following remarks are based largely on our collaborative research programme, based at the Gombe National Park in Tanzania and at Stanford University. Chimpanzee threat and attack patterns occur most often in these contexts: (1) When there is competition over food, especially if highly desirable foods are spatially concentrated or in short supply. (2) When an infant is being defended by its mother. (3) If a contest occurs over the dominance prerogatives of two individuals of similar social rank. (4) As a redirection of aggression: for example, when a low-ranking male has been attacked by a high-ranking male, it often turns to attack an individual subordinate to itself. (5) With failure of one animal to comply with a signal given by the aggressor: for example, when one chimpanzee does not respond to another's invitation to groom. (6) If one of the animals appears strange or different: for example, when the lower extremities of a chimpanzee became paralysed, it was attacked. (7) When changes in dominance status occur, over time, especially among the adolescent and young adult males. (8) During the formation of consort pairs at the peak of oestrus. (9) When relative strangers meet. (10) In the hunting and killing of small animals, such as infant baboon and infant colobus monkey.

It is possible, considering all the situations or conditions which elicit aggressive behaviour in chimpanzees, to group them largely into two categories, or to extract two themes from them: first, where protection is the issue and second, around access to valued resources.

In East Africa we have observed the common olive baboon in both savannah and forest habitats. In addition, one finds reports of similar observations by Hall (1965), DeVore (1965), Washburn (1968), Altman (1967), Rowell (1967), and Ransom (1971). From this work the main eliciting conditions of baboon threat and attack patterns can be summarized as follows: (1) When adult males are protecting the troop against predators, such as lions and

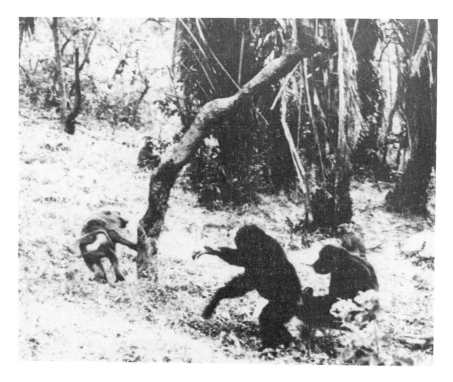

FIGURE 1 Chimp throws rock at baboon (photo: Eric Hamburg)

cheetahs. (2) In the protection of infants both by the mothers and adult males. (3) During resolution of disputes between adult males within the troop. (4) When consort pairs are being formed at the peak of oestrus. (5) For the attainment of preferred sleeping locations in the trees, particularly in the presence of predators. (6) When acquiring premium foods such as figs, nuts, and bananas, especially when they are spatially concentrated rather than widely distributed. (7) As part of dominance interactions, especially in the presence of premium foods, scarcity of sleeping sites, and females in full oestrus. (8) During the exploration of strange or manifestly dangerous areas, a function largely of adult males. (9) Where contact occurs between different troops, especially if such contact is infrequent.

In all of these circumstances the probability of overt threat behaviour, and of fighting, is higher than in the other contexts of baboon life. In baboons, as in chimpanzees, much of the day is spent in peaceful activities, and there is abundant evidence of affectional systems similar to those analysed

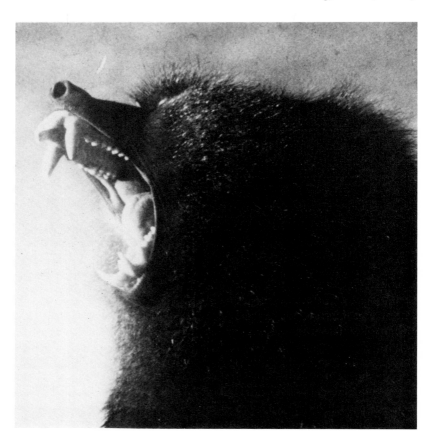

FIGURE 2 Baboon threat: canine display (photo: Eric Hamburg)

experimentally by Harlow in rhesus macaques. The popular question, therefore, as to whether monkeys and apes are peaceful or aggressive is scarcely
meaningful as a scientific question. They clearly show both kinds of
characteristics — sometimes they fight and sometimes they do not. We are
trying to clarify the conditions under which they are likely to threaten or
attack — that is, what circumstances appear to precipitate such behaviour.

It will be noted that the lists of situations eliciting threat and attack
patterns in chimpanzees and in baboons does *not* include the defence of a
fixed territory. Our observations are consistent with those of Crook (1968)
who said, 'Comparative studies of forest-fringe and savannah cercopithecus
and macaca monkeys, the baboons of the genera papio and theropithecus, the

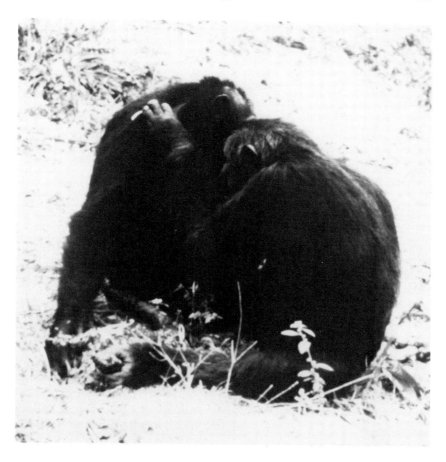

FIGURE 3 Adult chimps grooming (photo: Eric Hamburg)

chimpanzee and gorilla do not provide evidence of rigorously defended territories.'

To qualify this, it should be added that although most higher primates do not live in permanently fixed territories that they defend rigorously, there is nevertheless a behavioural distinction between currently familiar and relatively unfamiliar territory. The savannah baboon troop may live in an area of five to ten square miles for some weeks or months before moving to another nearby area. While it is living in a given area, the behaviour of its members tends to take on distinctive features at the fringes of this 'currently familiar space.' They appear highly vigilant, threaten readily, and some males move out a considerable distance beyond females and young in exploring the relatively unfamiliar area. Sometimes they come in contact with other similar groups of baboons. From the limited data available at present, there appears to be considerable caution, vigilance, and agonistic behaviour when groups meet, though usually they seem to avoid serious fighting. There are, however (Southwick, 1969) some conditions under which serious intergroup fighting does indeed occur. This may be seen, for example, among rhesus macaque groups in cities under conditions of crowding, food shortage, and interspecies harrassment. An important topic for future research would be contact between groups under different circumstances. There is a particularly pressing need for field studies that focus on intergroup relationships.

CONTROLS IN MAN

A fundamental and difficult question, on which such studies might shed some light, and to which it seems there are no good answers, concerns the use of ritual in man to discharge aggressive impulses. It has been said, with some sense, that there are some patterns like the smile that go across cultures and tend to have the effect of soothing a hostile impulse. Most of this, however, we try to do with language, and with language as an instrument of culture. If there are, as a student of evolution would view it, long periods of relatively stable environmental conditions, including stable cultural guidelines for behaviour, it would seem quite possible to internalize norms that regulate the expression of hostility between individuals and between groups. Since the industrial revolution, and particularly in this century, the rate of technological and concomitant social change has been so great that these guide-lines for behaviour are less clear and controlling than they have been at some other times. Therefore, these primarily verbally transmitted guidelines for behaviour, in the form of cultural norms, probably do not have the strength and regulating capacity that they would have under more stable environmental conditions. However, history shows that even when conditions within a culture are relatively stable for long periods, there is still a very great problem: the readiness with which our species seems able to learn in-group/out-group distinctions — sharp dichotomies with rather drastic depreciation of the out-group. In that kind of consideration, not only is hostility important, but a kind of altruism is also important. As Donald Campbell (1965) has pointed out, devotion to one's own group may be just as dangerous as hostility toward the other group — for example, in the willingness to die for one's own group or to massacre others in the name of some 'good' cause. These phenomena have been widely distributed in various times and various places. One of the most poignant dilemmas in this era is how it may ever be possible to achieve some regulation of that kind of inter-group hostility.

HORMONES AND AGGRESSION

Evolutionary considerations call attention to the possibility that man has a vertebrate, mammalian, primate heritage predisposing to aggressive behaviour. But what is known of the processes that govern the expression of such predispositions in the person — that is, in the individual life cycle? One area that has become quite important in the past decade concerns early hormonal influences upon brain organization affecting later aggressive and sexual behaviour. Pioneering work was done with rodents in this respect, and then extended to monkeys by Young, Goy, and Phoenix (1964) with the co-operation of Harlow. It has been demonstrated that the administration of a rather large dose of testosterone to a pregnant monkey during roughly the second quarter of gestation tends to masculinize a female fetus in some anatomical and behavioural respects — one of the behavioural effects being to make these females somewhat more aggressive than untreated females. Using reliable scoring systems it has been established that they engage more in rough-and-tumble play and initiate social threat more than females who have not been exposed to high levels of testosterone in utero. Of course, over the years of growth and development many influences can modify the expression of these aggressive patterns that have been influenced by testosterone. For example, undue infant aggressiveness in a female may be severely punished by larger and more powerful animals, leading to fearful inhibition later in life. In view of such considerations it is particularly interesting that there is some tendency toward persistence of these hyper-aggressive characteristics into adult life in the female monkeys whose mothers were exposed to testosterone in pregnancy.

One may well ask: Is there any evidence that testosterone may have similar effects on behaviour development in man? Some years ago when the findings in monkeys were first reported we accumulated some cases of androgen-exposure during pregnancy in humans, though too few for an adequate study. Fortunately, the pediatric endocrine clinic at Johns Hopkins has a resource, unique in the world, of endocrine variations. John Money has been conducting a long-term programme of research in that setting. He and Anke Ehrhardt (1968) have now studied twenty-five girls, mostly in late childhood and early adolescence, whose mothers had been exposed to androgens before their births. Those of them who, as newborns, had shown striking anatomical abnormalities underwent surgical correction shortly after birth. With interviews and projective tests, data were obtained from each girl, at least one parent and some other informants, in several behavioural categories. The research design undertook to control for observer bias. The results indicated that the early-androgenized girls, as contrasted with a control group, tended to be described by self and others as 'tomboys,' to engage in outdoor sports requiring much energy and vigour, to prefer rough play, and to prefer toys ordinarily chosen by boys – such as guns. Although this initial study will be difficult to replicate, every effort must be made to do so because of the importance of the findings. The results so far are at least compatible with the concept that testosterone is one of many influences shaping the development of aggressive behaviour in our own species.

LEARNING OF AGGRESSIVE PATTERNS

If these results are confirmed, does it mean that exposure of the fetal brain to testosterone has a distinctive influence on differentiation of circuits that will later mediate aggressive responses? That seems likely, in view of current research (Clayton, 1970) on biochemical mechanisms of brain differentiation. Testosterone does seem to have important effects on the developing brain at a molecular level. It would not, however, suggest that testosterone establishes fixed patterns of complex behaviour unmodifiable by subsequent events. More likely, the hormone affects the brain in a way that facilitates the learning of aggressive patterns later in life. For any species, some patterns of behaviour are easy to learn, some more difficult, and some exceedingly so. In general, patterns that have been valuable in species survival are easy to learn.

Hormonal influences on brain development may have important mediating roles, especially where sex differentiation is concerned. One way that this can occur is through differences in development of attention, since attention is crucial in learning processes. A hormonal influence during a sensitive period of brain development may render a certain class of stimuli more interesting to the organism at a later stage. This line of inquiry is amenable to experimental analysis in non-human primates and to a certain extent in human infants. The best model for this is an experiment by Sackett (1966) in the Wisconsin laboratories. He showed that isolation-reared rhesus macaques, exposed to various kinds of pictures, indicate certain preferences and certain distinctive reactions. One is that they tend to spend more time looking at monkey pictures than at non-monkey pictures. Another is that within the various classes of monkey stimuli there is a particularly powerful and emotionally-disturbing effect caused by the full-face threat – a species-typical aggressive expression. The full-face threat between two and four months of life in the macaque has a dramatic effect. It is not difficult to imagine (though it is by no means demonstrated) that once an infant has had its attention powerfully drawn to the full-face threat, it could readily go on to learn a great deal about the conditions under which threat occurs, the conditions under which it is likely to be carried on to attack, and the actions that will tend to ameliorate the threat. How would such learning occur?

This brings us to a consideration of observational learning in primate adaptation. Traditionally, the popular discussions of aggressive behaviour have associated unlearned responses with non-human animals. One of the most interesting findings (Hamburg, 1969) of primate field studies of the past decade has been the recurrent theme of observational learning in a social context. In many species and diverse habitats, a behavioural sequence has been described. It begins with close observation of one animal by another. This is followed by imitation by the observing animal of the behaviour of the observed animal. The third part of the sequence is practice of the observed behaviour, often even some hours after its occurrence, especially in the play group of young animals. This sequence (observation, imitation, practice) has been described in relation to several adaptive situations: food-getting, tool-using, tool-making in chimps, nest-building, infant care, copulation, and aggressive interactions. In essence, the young have access to virtually the full range of adult behaviour and seem to take advantage of it to learn patterns of behaviour that have been effective in adaptation. Moreover, in experimental studies (Riopelle, 1960) it has been shown that the observing animal learns from incorrect, as well as from correct, responses in the animal he is watching. In other words, he can learn from the consequence of the observed animal's mistakes.

The above field observations are consistent with two concepts, though much more research is needed to establish these concepts firmly: (1) Aggressive patterns may be learned early in life through observation-imitation-practice sequences. (2) There is a sex difference in the attractiveness of some aggressive patterns from infancy onward, with males generally tending to be more interested and spending more time in practising the aggressive patterns.

It would appear that non-human primate data are very provocative with respect to future lines of inquiry in child development. To some extent work has already been done that indicates the direction such inquiry might take. The series of experiments by Bandura (1965) and his colleagues at Stanford over a number of years on observational learning in nursery school children have shown how remarkably ready they are to learn aggressive patterns by observing models who behave aggressively. So, although the scientific study of aggressive behaviour is relatively new and on a small scale, there are some promising lines of inquiry. Above all, what we need, and have rarely achieved, is an effective conjunction of the biological and psychosocial disciplines in tackling problems of aggression.

DEDICATION

Clarence Meredith Hincks, BA, MD, DSc, LLD
1885-1964

Born in St Mary's, Ontario, in 1885, Clarence Hincks was influenced in his formative years by a family vocational tradition exemplified by his mother, who was a teacher, and his father, who was a clergyman. He was graduated from the University of Toronto medical school in 1907 and became interested in psychiatry after some time in practice.

In 1918, with the support of Dr C.K. Clarke and Clifford Beer, he founded the Canadian National Committee for Mental Hygiene which was later to become the Canadian Mental Health Association. He is also remembered for his energetic and progressive involvement in many other aspects of the mental health field. Over half a century he worked to better the lot of the mentally ill through improved facilities and more enlightened treatment approaches. His influence on Canadian and international psychiatry was substantial, as he crusaded for better teaching programmes and research, partly through closer liaison with the social sciences.

In 1965, the Ontario Mental Health Foundation established an annual lectureship in honour of the late Dr Hincks. Its purpose was to stimulate workers in psychiatry and related disciplines by promoting the exchange of ideas and offering a platform for distinguished thinkers in the field. The present volume, very much in the spirit of Dr Hincks's lifelong interests and concerns, is the outcome of the third annual realization of this plan.

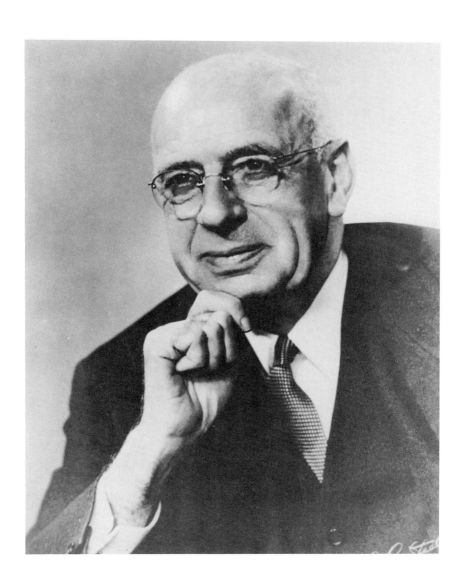

BIBLIOGRAPHY

NORMAN F. WHITE

Ethology and Psychiatry

Ainsworth, M.D. 1962. The effects of maternal deprivation: a review of findings and controversy in the context of research strategy. In *Deprivation of Maternal Care: A Reassessment of Its Effects*. Geneva: WHO public health papers, no. 14, 97-165

Altmann, S.A. 1967. The structure of primate social communication. In S.A. Altmann (ed.) *Social Communication Among Primates*. Chicago: University of Chicago Press

Ambrose, J.A. 1963. The concept of a critical period for the development of social responsiveness in early human infancy. In B.M. Foss, *Determinants of Infant Behavior (II)*. London: Methuen

Ambrose, J.A. 1968. The comparative approach to early child development: the data of ethology. In E. Miller (ed.), *Foundations of Child Psychiatry*. Oxford: Pergamon

Andrew, R.J. 1963. Evolution of facial expression. *Science* 142, 1034-41

Ardrey, R. 1961. *African Genesis*. London: Collins

Ardrey, R. 1966. *The Territorial Imperative*. New York: Atheneum

Arling, G.L. and Harlov, H.F. 1967. *J.Comp.Physiol.*, 64, 371-7

Barker, R.G. 1968. *Ecological Psychology – Concepts and Methods for Studying the Environment of Human Behavior*. Stanford, California: Stanford University Press

Barnett, S.A. 1955. 'Displacement' behavior and 'psychosomatic' disorder. *Lancet* 1203-8

Barnett, S.A. 1961. The behavior and needs of infant mammals. *Ibid.* 1067-71

Barnett, S.A. 1962. Attitudes to childhood. In S.A. Barnett (ed.), *Lessons from Animal Behavior for the Clinician*. (National Spastics Society.) London: Heinemann

Barnett, S.A. 1963. *A Study in Animal Behavior*. London: Methuen

Barnett, S.A. 1964. The biology of aggression. *Lancet* (Oct. 10), 803-7

Barnett, S.A. 1968. The 'instinct to teach.' *Nature* 220 (Nov. 23), 747-9

Bastian, J. 1965. Primate signalling systems and human languages. In I. DeVore (ed.), *Primate Behavior: Field Studies of Monkeys and Apes*. New York: Holt, Rinehart and Winston

Beach, F.A. 1955. The descent of instinct. *Psychol. Rev.* 62, 401-10

Beer, C.G. 1963. Ethology – the zoologist's approach to behavior, I. *Tuatara* 11, 170-7

Beer, C.G. 1964. Ethology – the zoologists's approach to behavior, II; *Tuatara* 12, 16-39

Beer, C.G. 1968. Ethology on the couch. In J.H. Masserman (ed.), *Animal and Human.* (*Science and Psychoanalysis,* vol. XII.) Scientific proceedings of the American Academy of Psychoanalysis. New York: Grune and Stratton

Berkowitz, L. 1962. *Aggression: A Social Psychological Analysis.* New York: McGraw-Hill

Birch, H.G. 1961. The pertinence of animal investigations for a science of human behavior. *Amer. J. Orthopsychiat.* 31, 267-75

Birdwhistell, R.L. 1959. Contribution of linguistic-kinesic studies to the understanding of schizophrenia. In A. Auerback (ed.), *Schizophrenia.* New York: Ronald

Blurton-Jones, N.G. 1967. An ethological study of some aspects of social behavior of children in nursery school. In D. Morris (ed.), *Primate Ethology.* Chicago: Aldine

Bowlby, J. 1951. *Maternal Care and Mental Health.* Geneva: WHO monograph series, no. 2

Bowlby, J. 1957. An ethological approach to research in child development. *Brit. J. Med. Psychol.* 30, 230-40

Bowlby, J. 1958. The nature of the child's tie to the mother. *Int. J. Psychoanal.* 39, 350-73

Bowlby, J. 1960. Ethology and the development of object relations. *Ibid.* 41, 313-7

Bowlby, J. 1960a. Grief and mourning in early infancy and early childhood. *Psychoanal. Stud. Child.* 15, 9-32

Bridger, W.H. 1963. Ethological concepts and human development. In J. Wortis (ed.), *Recent Advances in Biological Psychiatry.* New York: Plenum

Brody, S. and Axelrad, S. 1966. *Anxiety, Socialization, and Ego Formation in Infancy.* New York: International Universities Press, Inc.

Bronfenbrenner, U. 1968. Early deprivation in mammals: a cross-species analysis. In G. Newton, and S. Levine, *Early Experience and Behavior.* Springfield: Charles Thomas

Bronson, G.W. 1962. Critical periods in human development. *Brit. J. Med. Psychol.* 35, 127-33

Bronson, G.W. 1965. The hierarchical organization of the central nervous system: implications for learning processes and critical periods in early development. *Behav. Sci.* 10, 7-26

Bronson, G.W. 1968. The development of fear in man and other animals. *Ch. Devel.* 39, 409-31

Brosin, H.W. 1960. Evolution and understanding diseases of the mind. In S. Tax (ed.), *Evolution After Darwin.* vol. II: *The Evolution of Man.* Chicago: University of Chicago Press

Brown, J.W. 1967. Physiology and phylogenesis of emotional expression. *Brain Research* 5, 1-14

Caldwell, B.M. 1968. The Social Biology of Human Beings. In R.E. Cooke (ed.), *The Biologic Basis of Pediatric Practice.* New York: McGraw-Hill

Campbell, B.G. 1966. *Human Evolution: An Introduction to Man's Adaptations.* Chicago: Aldine

Carpenter, C.R. 1964. Territoriality: a review of concepts and problems. In C.R. Carpenter, *Naturalistic Behavior of Nonhuman Primates.* University Park, Pa.: Pennsylvania State University Press

Carthy, J.D., and Ebling, F.J. (eds.). 1964. *The Natural History of Aggression*. London: Academic Press

Casler, L. 1961. Material deprivation: a critical review of the literature. *Monogr. Soc. Res. Child Develop.* 26, No. 2

Clemente, C. and Lindsley, D. (eds.), 1967. *Aggression and Defense: Neural Mechanisms and Social Patterns*. Los Angeles: University California Press

Colman, A.D. 1968. Territoriality in man: a comparison of behavior in home and hospital. *Am. J. Orthopsychiat.* 38, 464-8

Craig, W. 1918. Appetites and aversions as constituents of instincts. *Biol. Bull.* 34, 91-107

Crook, J.H. 1970. Social behavior and ethology. In J.H. Crook (ed.), *Social Behavior in Birds and Mammals: Essays on the Social Ethology of Animals and Man*. New York: Academic Press

Crook, J.H. 1970a. Social organization and the environment: aspects of contemporary social ethology. *Anim. Behav.* 18, 197-209

Crook, J.H. and Gartlan, J.S. 1966. Evolution of primate societies. *Nature* 210, 1200-3

Daniels, D.M., Gilvla, M.F. and Ochberg, F.M. 1970. *Violence and the Struggle for Existence*. Boston: Little, Brown

Darwin, C.R. 1859. *The Origin of Species*. New York: Appleton

Darwin, C.R. 1871. *The Descent of Man*. New York: Appleton

Darwin, C.R. 1872. *The Expression of Emotions in Man and Animals*. London: Murray

Davis, D.E. 1962. An inquiry into the phylogeny of gangs. In E.L. Bliss (ed.), *Roots of Behavior*. New York: Harper

Demaret, A. 1971. Essai d'explication de l'anorexie mentale de la jeune fille dans la perspective ethologique. *Acta psychiat. belg.* 71, 5-23

Diamond, M. 1965. A critical evaluation of the ontogeny of human sexual behavior. *Quart. Rev. Biol.* 40, 147-75

Dolhinow, P. 1971. At play in the fields. *Nat. Hist. Bio.* 80 (10), 66-71

Drewe, E.A., Ettlinger, G., Milner, A.D., and Passingham, R.E. 1970. A comparative review of the results of neurophysiological research on man and monkey. *Cortex* 6, 129-63

Eibl-Eibesfeldt, I. 1967. Concepts of ethology and their significance on the study of human behavior. In H.W. Stevenson (ed.), *Early Behavior: Comparative and Development Approaches*. New York: Wiley, 127-46

Eibl-Eibesfeldt, I. 1970. *Ethology – The Biology of Behavior*. New York: Holt, Rinehart and Winston

Eibl-Eibesfeldt, I. and Kramer, S. 1958. Ethology and the comparative study of animal behavior. *Quart. Rev. Biol.* 33 (3), 181-211

Eisenberg, L. 1972. The *human* nature of human nature. *Science* 176, 4031 (April 14, 1972), 123-8

Engel, G.L. 1969. Psychological factors in ulcerative colitis in man and Gibbon. *Gastroenterology* 57, 362-5

Esser, A. 1965. Social contact and the use of space in psychiatric patients. *Amer. Zool.* 5, 231

Esser, A.H. 1971. *Behavior and Environment. The Use of Space by Animals and Man*. New York: Renum

Esser, A., Chamberlain, A., Chapple, E., and Kline, N., 1965. Territoriality of patients on a research ward. *Rec. Adv. Biol. Psychiat.* 7, 37-44

Esser, A., and Poluck, R. 1968. Dominance hierarchy and clinical course of psychiatrically hospitalized boys. *Child Develop.* 39, 147-57

Ewer, R.F. 1968. *Ethology of Mammals.* New York: Plenum Press

Fletcher, R. 1957. *Instinct in Man: In the Light of Recent Work in Comparative Psychology.* London: Allen and Unwin

Fox, M.W. 1968. Aggression: its adaptive and maladaptive significance in man and animals. In M.W. Fox, *Abnormal Behavior in Animals.* Philadelphia: Saunders

Fox, M.W. 1968a. Ethology: an overview. In Fox, *Abnormal Behavior in Animals*

Fox, R. 1967. In the beginning: aspects of hominid behavioral evolution. *Man* 2, 415-33

Frank, R.L. 1954. The organized adaptive aspect of the depression-elation response. In P.H. Hoch and J. Zubin (eds.), *Depression.* New York: Grune and Stratton

Freedman, D.G. 1965. An ethological approach to the genetical study of human behavior. In S. Vandenburg (ed.), *Methods and Goals in Human Behavior Genetics* New York: Academic Press

Freedman, D.G. 1968. Personality development in infancy: a biological approach. In S.L. Washburn and P.C. Jay (eds.), *Perspectives on Human Evolution.* New York: Holt, Rinehart and Winston.

Freedman, D.G., King, J.A., and Elliot, E. 1961. Critical period in the social development of dogs. *Science* 133, 1016-17

Garrattini, S. and Sigg, E. (eds.). 1969. *Aggressive Behavior.* New York: Wiley

Graham, M. 1964. Crowds and the like in vertebrates. *Hum. Rel.* 17, 377-90

Grant, E.C. 1965. The contribution of ethology to child psychiatry. In J.G. Howells (ed.), *Modern Perspectives in Child Psychiatry.* Edinburgh: Oliver and Boyd

Grant, E.C. 1965a. An ethological description of some schizophrenic patterns of behavior. *Proc. Leeds Symposium on Behavioral Disorders,* chap. 12. Dagenham, Essex, England: May and Baker Ltd

Grant, E.C. 1968. An ethological description of non-verbal behavior during interviews. *Brit. J. Med. Psychol.* 41, 177-83

Gray, P.H. 1958. Theory and evidence of imprinting in human infants. *J. Psychol.* 46, 155-66

Griffin, G.A. and Harlow, H.F. 1966. Effects of three months of total social deprivation on social adjustment and learning in the rhesus monkey. *Child Develop.* 37, 533-47

Haeckel, E. 1910. *The Evolution of Man* (trans. Joseph McCabe). London: Watts

Haldane, J.B.S. 1953. Animal ritual and human language. *Diogenes* 1 (4), 61-73

Haldane, J.B.S. 1955. Animal communication and the origin of human language. *Sci. Prog.* 43, 385-401

Hall, E.T. 1959. *The Silent Language.* New York: Doubleday

Hall, E.T. 1966. *The Hidden Dimension.* New York: Doubleday

Hamburg, D.A. 1962. The relevance of recent evolutionary changes to human stress biology. In S. Washburn (ed.), *Social Life of Early Man.* Chicago: Aldine

Hamburg, D.A. 1968. Emotions in the perspective of human evolution. In
S.L. Washburn and P.C. Jay (eds.), *Perspectives on Human Evolution I.*
New York: Holt, Rinehart, Winston

Hamburg, D.A. 1968a. Evolution of emotional responses: evidence from
recent research on nonhuman primates. In Masserman (ed.), *Animal and
Human.* (*Science and Psychoanalysis,* vol. II)

Hampson, J.L. and Hampson, J.G. 1961. The ontogenesis of sexual behavior
in man. In W.C. Young (ed.), *Sex and Internal Secretions.* Baltimore:
Williams and Wilkins

Harlow H.F. 1959. Love in infant monkeys. *Sci. Am.* (June 1959), 68-74

Harlow, H.F. 1963. The maternal affectional system. In B.M. Foss (ed.), *The
Determinants of Infant Behavior,* 3-33. New York: Wiley

Harlow, H.F., Dodsworth, R.O., and Harlow, M.K. 1965. Total social isolation in monkeys. *Proc. Nat. Acad. Sci.* 54, 90-7

Harlow, H.F. and Harlow, M.K. 1962. Social deprivation in monkeys. *Sci.
Am.* 2-7, 137-46

Harlow, H.F. and Harlow, M.K. 1965. The affectional systems. In A.M.
Schrier, H.F. Harlow and F. Stollnitz (eds.), *Behavior of Nonhuman
Primates, Vol. 2,* 287-334. New York: Academic Press

Harlow, H.F. and Suomi, S.J. 1970. Induced psychopathology in monkeys.
Engineering and Science 33, 8-14

Harlow, H.F., Suomi, S.J., and McKinney, W.T. 1970. Experimental production of depression in monkeys. *Mainly Monkeys* 1, 6-12

Harlow, H.F. and Suomi, S.J. 1971. Production of depressive behaviours in
young monkeys. *J. Aut. Ch. Schiz.* 1 (3), 246-55

Hebb, D.O. 1953. Heredity and environment in mammalian behavior. *Brit. J.
Anim. Behav.* I, 43-7

Hebb, D.O. and Thompson, W.R. 1954. The social significance of animal
studies. In *Handbook of Social Psychology,* vol. I: *Theory and Method.*
Reading, Mass.: Addison-Wesley Publishing Company, Inc

Hediger, H.P. 1961. The evolution of territorial behavior. In Washburn, *Social
Life of Early Man*

Heinroth, O. 1910. Beitrage zur Biologie, namentlich Ethologie und
Physiologie der Anatiden. 5. *International Ornith. Verh. 5,* 589-702

Hess, E.H. 1959. Imprinting. *Science* (July 17), 130-41

Hess, E.H. 1962. Ethology: an approach toward the complete analysis of
behavior. In R. Brown et al., *New Directions in Psychology* 157-266. New
York: Holt, Rinehart, and Winston

Hess, E.H. 1967. Ethology. In A.M. Freedman and H.I. Kaplan (eds.), *Com-
perhensive Textbook of Psychiatry.* Baltimore: Williams and Wilkins

Hess, E.H. 1970. Ethology and developmental psychology. In P.H. Mussen
(ed.), *Manual of Child Psychology,* Vol. 1, chap. 1, 1-38. New York: Wiley

Hewes, G.H. 1957. The anthropology of posture. *Sci. Am.* 196, 123-32

Hinde, R.A. 1956. Ethological models and the concept of 'drive.' *Brit. J. Phil.
Sci.* 6, 321

Hinde, R.A. 1959. Unitary drives. *Anim. Behav.* 7, 130-41

Hinde, R.A. 1960. Energy models of motivation. *Symp. Exp. Biol.* 14, 199-213

Hinde, R.A. 1962. Sensitive periods and the development of behavior. In S.A.
Barnett (ed.), *Lessons from Animal Behavior for the Clinician* (National
Spastics Society). London: Heinemann

Hinde, R.A. 1962a. The relevance of animal studies to human neurotic disorders. In C.P. Richter (ed.), *Aspects of Psychiatric Research*. Oxford: Oxford University Press

Hinde, R.A. 1967. The nature of aggression. *New Society* 9 (March 1967), 302-4

Hinde, R.A. 1969. Analyzing the roles of the partners in a behavioral interaction in mother-infant relations in rhesus macaques. *Ann. N.Y. Acad. Sci.* 159, 651-67

Hinde, R.A. 1969a. The bases of aggression in animals. *J. Psychosom. Res.* 13, 213-19

Hinde, R.A. 1970. *Animal Behaviour: A Synthesis of Ethology and Comparative Psychology*. 2nd ed. New York: McGraw-Hill

Hinde, R.A. and Atkinson, S. 1970a. Assessing the roles of social partners in maintaining mutual proximity, as exemplified by mother-infant relations in rhesus monkeys. *Anim. Behav.* 18, 169-76

Hinde, R.A. and Spencer-Booth, Y. 1967a. The effect of social companions on mother-infant relations in infant monkeys. In D. Morris (ed.), *Primate Ethology*. Chicago: Aldine

Hinde, R.A. and Spencer-Booth, Y. 1971. Effects of brief separation from mother on rhesus monkeys. *Science* 173, 111-18

Hinde, R.A. and Tinbergen, N. 1958. The comparative study of species-specific behaviour. In A. Roe and C.G. Simpson (eds.), *Behavior and Evolution*. New Haven: Yale

Hockett, C.F. 1960. The origin of speech. *Sci. Am.* 203, 89-96

Horowitz, M. 1968. Spatial behavior and psychopathology. *J. Nerv. Ment. Dis.* 168, 24-35

Hutt, C., Hutt, S.J., and Oustead, C. 1963. A method for the study of children's behavior. *Develop. Med. Child Neurol.* 5, 233-45

Imanishi, K. 1965. Identification: a process of socialization in the subhuman society of *Macaca fuscata*. In S.A. Altmann (ed.), *Japanese Monkeys – A Collection of Translations*. Edmonton, Alberta: Department of Zoology, University of Alberta

Imanishi, K. 1965a. The origin of the human family – a primatological approach. In Altmann (ed.), *Japanese Monkeys – A Collection of Translations*.

Jaynes, J. 1969. The historical origins of 'ethology' and 'comparative psychology.' *Anim. Behav.* 17, 601-6

Jensen, G.D. and Bobbitt, R.A. 1968. Implications of primate research for understanding infant development. In Masserman (ed.), *Animal and Human. (Science and Psychoanalysis,* vol. XII*)*

Jensen, G.D. and Tolman, C.W. 1962. Mother-infant relationship in the monkey, *Macaca Venestrina:* the effect of brief separation and mother-infant specificity. *J. Comp. Physiol. Psychol.* 55, 1, 131-6

Kaufman, I.C. 1960a. Some ethological studies of social relationships and conflict situations. *J. Am. Psychoan. Ass.* 8, 671-85

Kaufman, I.C. 1960a. Some theoretical implications from animal behavior studies for the psycho-analytic concepts of instinct, energy, and drive. *Int. J. Psychoan.* 41, 318-26

Kaufman, I.C. 1970. Biologic considerations of parenthood. In E.J. Anthony and T. Benedek, *Parenthood: Its Psychology and Psychopathology*. Boston: Little, Brown

Kaufman, I.C. and Rosenblum, L.A. 1967. Depression in infant monkeys separated from their mothers. *Science* 155, 1030-1

Kaufman, I.C. and Rosenblum, L.A. 1967a. The reaction to separation in infant monkeys: anaclitic depression and conservation-withdrawal. *Psychosom. Med.* 29, 648-75

Kaufman, I.C. and Rosenblum, L.A. 1969. Effects of separation from mother on the emotional behavior of infant monkeys. *Ann. N.Y. Acad. Scie.* 159, 681-95

Klopfer, P.H. and Hailman, J.P. 1967. *An Introduction to Animal Behavior: Ethology's First Century.* Englewood Cliffs, NJ: Prentice-Hall

Kortmulder, K. 1968. An ethological theory of the incest taboo and exogamy. *Curr. Anthropol.* 9 (5), 437-49

Kramer, S. 1968. Fixed motor patterns in ethologic and psychoanalytic theory. In Masserman (ed.), *Animal and Human.* (*Science and Psychoanalysis*, vol. XII)

Kraus, R.F. 1970. Implications of recent developments in primate research for psychiatry. *Comp. Psychiat,* II (4), 528-35

Kuhme, W. 1963. Ergänzende Beobachtungen an afrikanischen Elefanten im Freigehege. *Z. Tierpsychol.* 20, 66-79

Kummer, Hans. 1971. *Societies: Group Techniques of Ecological Adaptation.* Chicago: Aldine

Lancaster, J.B. 1966. Primate communication systems and the emergence of human language. In P. Jay (ed.), *Primate Social Behavior.* New York: Holt, Rinehart, Winston

Lehrman, D.S. 1953. A critique of Konrad Lorenz's theory of instinctive behavior. *Quarterly Review of Biology* 28 (4), 337-63

Lehrman, D.S. 1963. Ethology and psychology. *Rec. Adv. Biol. Psychiat.* 4, 86-94

Leyhausen, P. 1956. Verhaltensstudien bei Katzen. *Z. Tierpsychol., Bieheft,* 2 (illustrations reprinted in Hinde, 1966)

Loizos, C. 1967. Play behavior in higher primates: a review. In D. Morris, *Primate Ethology.* Chicago: Aldine

Lorenz, K. 1952. *King Solomon's Ring.* London: Methuen

Lorenz, K. 1953. Die Entwicklung der vergleichenden Verhaltenforschung in den letzten 12 Jahren. *Verh. dtsch. Zool. Ges. Freiburg* 1952, 36-58 (quoted in Eibl-Eibesfeldt and Kramer, 1958)

Lorenz, K. 1958. The evolution of behavior. *Sci. Am.* 199, 67-78

Lorenz, K. 1963. *On Aggression.* New York: Harcourt, Brace and World, Inc

Lorenz, K. 1965. *Evolution and Modification of Behavior.* Chicago: University of Chicago Press

Lorenz, K. 1970. The enmity between generations and its probably ethological causes. *Stud. Gen.* 23, 963-97

Lorenz, K. 1971. Der Mensch, biologischgesenen. *Stud. Gen.* 24, 495-515

Manning, A. 1967. *An Introduction to Animal Behaviour.* London: Edward Arnold

Marks, I. 1971. *Fears and Phobias.* New York: Academic Press

Marler, P. and Hamilton, W.J. 1966. *Mechanisms of Animal Behaviour.* New York: Wiley

Mason, W.A. 1968. Early social deprivation in the nonhuman primates: implications for human behavior. In D.C. Glass (ed.), *Environmental Influences.* New York: Rockefeller University Press and Russell Sage Foundation

Mason, W.A., 1968a. Scope and potential of primate research. In Masserman (ed.), *Animal and Human. (Science and Psychoanalysis,* vol. XII*)*

Mason, W.A. and Riopelle, A.J. 1964. Comparative psychology. *Ann. Rev. Psychol.* 15, 143-80

Masserman, J.H. 1968. Comparative and clinical approaches to biodynamic therapy. In Masserman (ed.), *Animal and Human. (Science and Psychoanalysis,* vol. XII*)*

McKinney, W.T. and Bunney, W.E. 1969. Animal model of depression. I. Review of evidence: implications for research. *Arch. Gen. Psychiat.* 21, 240-8

McKinney, W.T., Suomi, S.J., and Harlow, H.F. 1971. Depression in primates. *Amer. J. Psychiat.* 127 (10) 1313-20

MacLean, P.D. 1973. *A Triune Concept of the Brain and Behaviour* Toronto: University of Toronto Press

Menaker, E. 1956. A note on some biologic parallels between certain innate animal behaviors and moral masochism. *Psychoanal. Rev.* 43, 31

Mill, J.S. 1843. Psychology and ethology. In *A System of Logic* (book six), chap. 3. In Dennis (ed.), *Readings in the History of Psychology.* New York: Appleton-Century-Crofts, 1948

Mitchell, W.M. 1969. Observations on animal behavior and its relationship to masochism. *Dis. Nerv. Syst.* 30, 124-9

Moltz, H. 1963. The fixed action pattern: empirical properties and theoretical implications. *Rec. Adv. Biol. Psychiat.* 4, 60-85

Money, J. 1965. Psychosexual differentiation. In J. Money, *Sex Research: New Developments.* New York: Holt, Rinehart, Winston

Montagu, M. (ed.). 1968. *Man and Aggression.* New York: Oxford University Press

Morgan, C.L. 1896. *Habit and Instinct.* London: Edward Arnold

Morris, D. (ed.). 1967. *Primate Ethology.* Chicago: Aldine

Morris, D. 1967a. *The Naked Ape.* New York: McGraw-Hill

Morris, D. 1969. *The Human Zoo.* New York: McGraw-Hill

Morris, D. 1971. *Intimate Behavior.* Toronto: Clarke Irwin

Morton, J. 1972. Man, the ritual animal. *Aust. N.Z. J. Psychiat.* 6, 133

Moses, L. 1968. The evolution of human behavior. In Masserman (ed.), *Animal and Human. (Science and Psychoanalysis,* vol. XII*)*

Moses, L. 1968a. An evolutionary-adaptational-ecologic view of human behavior. In Masserman (ed.), *Animal and Human. (Science and Psychoanalysis,* vol. XII*)*

O'Connor, N. 1968. Children in restricted environments. In G. Newton and S. Levine, *Early Experience and Behavior.* Springfield: Chas. Thomas

Ostow, M. 1959. The structural model: Ego, id, and superego. *Ann. N.Y. Acad. Sci.* 76, 1098-134

Ostow, M. 1960. Psychoanalysis and ethology. *J. Am. Psychoan. Ass.,* 8, 526-34

Pfeiffer, J.E. 1969. *The Emergence of Man.* New York: Harper and Row

Pivnicki, D. 1970. Aggression reconsidered. In F.A. Freyhan (ed.), *Comprehensive Psychiatry,* vol. XI. New York and London: Henry M. Stratton, Inc

Price, J.S. 1967. The dominance hierarchy and the evolution of mental illness. *Lancet* (July 29), 243-6

Price, J.S. 1969. The ritualization of agonistic behavior as a determinant of variation along the neuroticism/stability dimension of personality. *Proc. Roy. Soc. Med.* 62, 1107-10

Reynolds, V. 1966. Open groups in hominid evolution. *Man* 1, 441-52

Roe, A. and Simpson, C.G. (eds.). 1958. *Behavior and Evolution.* New Haven: Yale

Roffwarg, H.P., Muzio, J.N., and Dement, W.C. 1966. Ontogenetic development of the human sleep-dream cycle. *Science* 152, 604-19

Romanes, G.J. 1884. *Mental Evolution in Animals.* London: Kegan, Paul, Trench

Romanes, G.J. 1889. *Mental Evolution in Man.* New York: Appleton

Rosenblatt, J.S. 1969. The development of maternal responsiveness in the rat. *Am. J. Orthopsychiat.* 39, 36-56

Rosenblum, L.A. and Kaufman, I.C. 1968. Variations in infant development and response to maternal loss in monkeys. *Am. J. Orthopsychiat.* 38, 418-26

Roth, L.H. 1971. Territoriality and homosexuality in a male prison population. *Ibid.* 41 (3) (April 1971), 510-13

Ruesch, J. 1953. Synopsis of the theory of human communication. *Psychiatry* 16, 215-43

Russell, C. and Russell, W.M.S. 1961. *Human Behavior, a New Approach.* New York: Little, Brown

Rutter, M. 1972. Maternal deprivation reconsidered. *J. Psychosom. Res.* 16, 241-50

Scheflen, A.E. 1963. Communication and regulation in psychotherapy. *Psychiatry* 26, 126

Schmale, A.H. 1964. A genetic view of affects with special reference to the genesis of helplessness and hopelessness. *Psychoanal. Stud. Child.* 19, 287-310

Schmidbauer, W. 1971. 'Methodenprobleme der Human-Ethologie. *Stud. Gen.* 24, 462-94

Schmidbauer, W. 1971a. 'Methodenprobleme der Human-Ethologie' — 'Der Mensch, biologischgesehen, *Ibid.* 516-22

Schneirla, T.C. and Rosenblatt, J.S. 1961. Behavioral organization and genesis of the social bond in insects and mammals. *Am. J. Orthopsychiat.* 31, 223-53

Schur, M. 1960. Discussion of Dr John Bowlby's paper. *Psychoanal. Stud. Child.* 15, 63-84

Schur, M. 1961. Animal research panel. (4) Discussion: a psychoanalyst's comments. *Am. J. Orthopsychiat.* 31, 276-91

Scott, J.P. 1958. *Aggression.* Chicago: University of Chicago Press

Scott, J.P. 1962. Genetics and the development of social behavior in mammals. *Am. J. Orthopsychiat.* 32, 878-93

Scott, J.P. 1962a. Hostility and aggression in animals. In E.L. Bliss (ed.), *Roots of Behavior.* New York: Harper

Scott, J.P. 1963. The process of primary socialization in canine and human infants. *Monogr. Soc. Res. Child Develop.* 28 (1), 1-47

Scott, J.P. 1969. The social psychology of infrahuman animals. In G. Lindzey, and E. Aronson, *The Handbook of Social Psychology.* Don Mills, Ontario: Addison-Wesley

Scott, J.P. 1970. Biology and human aggression. *Am. J. Orthopsychiat.* 40, 568-76

Seay, B., Hansen, E., and Harlow, H.F. 1962. Mother-infant separation in monkeys. *J. Child Psychol. Psychiat.* 3, 123-32

Seay, B. and Harlow, H.F. 1965. Maternal separation in the rhesus monkey. *J. Nerv. Ment. Dis.* 140, 434

Sebeok, T.A. 1965. Animal communication. *Science* 147, 1006-14

Simpson, G.G. 1966. The biological nature of man. *Ibid.* 152, 472-8

Slater, M.K. 1968. Primate parallels and bio-cultural models. In Masserman (ed.), *Animal and Human. (Science and Psychoanalysis,* vol. XII*)*

Sluckin, W. 1964. *Imprinting and Early Learning.* London: Methuen

Snyder, F. 1966. Toward an evolutionary theory of dreaming. *Amer. J. Psychiat.* 123, 121-36

Spencer-Booth, Y. and Hinde, R.A. 1907. The effects of separating rhesus monkey infants from their mothers for six days. *J. Child Psychol. Psychiat.* 7, 179-97

Spitz, R.A. 1946. Anaclitic depression. *Psychoanal. Stud. Child.* 2, 313-47

Storr, A. 1968. *Human Aggression.* London: Allen Lane

Suomi, S.J. and Harlow, H.F. 1971. Monkeys at play. *Nat. Hist.* 80 (10), 72-5

Suomi, S.J. and Harlow, H.F. 1972. Depressive behavior in young monkeys subjected to vertical chamber confinement. *J. Comp. Physiol. Psychol.* 180 (1), 11-18

Suomi, S.J., Harlow, H.F., and Domek, C.J. 1970. Effects of repetitive infant-infant separation of young monkeys. *J. Abn. Psychol.* 76 (2), 161-72

Taketomo, Y. 1968. The application of imprinting to psychodynamics. In Masserman (ed.), *Animal and Human. (Science and Psychoanalysis,* vol. XII*)*

Thorpe, W.H. 1956. Ethology as a new branch of biology. An A.A. Buzzati-Traverso, *Perspectives in Marine Biology.* Berkeley: University California Press. Reprinted in McGill, T.E. 1965. *Readings in Animal Behavior.* New York: Holt, Rinehart, Winston

Thorpe, W.H. 1956a. *Learning and Instinct in Animals.* London: Methuen

Tiger, L. 1969. *Men in Groups.* New York: Random House

Tiger, L. and Fox, R. 1966. The zoological perspective in social science. *Man* 1 (1) (March), 75

Tinbergen, N. 1951. *The Study of Instinct.* London: Clarendon Press

Tinbergen, N. 1963. On aims and methods of ethology. *Z. Tierpsychol.* 20, 410-33

Tinbergen, N. 1968. On war and peace in animals and man. *Science* 160, 1411-18

Tobach, E. and Schneirla, T. 1968. Biopsychology of social behavior in animals. In R.E. Cooke (ed.), *Biologic Basis of Pediatric Practice.* New York: McGraw-Hill

Uexkull, J. von. 1909. *Umwelt und Innenwelt der Tiere.* Berlin: Springer-Verlag

Vaughan, V.C. 1966. New insights in social behavior. *JAMA* 198, 163-6

Whitman, C.O. 1919. The behavior of pigeons. *Carnegie Inst. of Wash. Pub.* 257, 1-161

Wickler, W. 1967. Socio-sexual signals and their intra-specific imitation among primates. In Morris (1967)

Wood-Gush, D.G.M. 1963. Comparative psychology and ethology. *Ann. Rev. Psychol.* 14, 175-200

Yarrow, A.J. and Goodwin, M.S. 1965. Some conceptual issues in the study of mother-infant interactions. *Am. J. Orthopsychiat.* 35, 473-81
Zegans, L.S. 1967. An appraisal of ethological contributions to psychiatric theory and research. *Am. J. Psychiat.* 124 (6), 37-47

ROBERT A. HINDE

1 Mother/Infant Relations in Rhesus Monkeys

Ardrey, R. 1967. *The Territorial Imperative: A Personal Inquiry into the Animal Origins of Property and Nations.* London: Collins

Bowlby, J. 1969. *Attachment and Loss.* vol. I: *Attachment.* London: Hogarth Press

Harlow, H.F. and Harlow, M.K. 1965. The affectional systems, in A.M. Schrier, H.F. Harlow, and F. Stollnitz (eds.), *Behaviour of Nonhuman Primates,* vol. II. New York: Academic Press

Hinde, R.A. 1969. Analyzing the roles of the partners in a behavioural interaction — mother/infant relations in rhesus macaques. *Ann. NY Acad. Sci.* 159, 651-667

Hinde, R.A. and Spencer-Booth, Y. 1967. The behaviour of socially living rhesus monkeys in their first two-and-a-half years. *Anim. Behav.* 15, 169-96

Hinde, R.A. and Spencer-Booth, Y. 1968. The study of mother/infant interaction in captive group-living rhesus monkeys. *Proc. Roy. Soc. B* 169, 177-201

Hinde, R.A. and Spencer-Booth, Y. Forthcoming. Towards understanding individual differences in rhesus mother-infant interaction. *Anim. Behav.*

Hinde, R.A. and Spencer-Booth, Y. Forthcoming. Individual differences in the responses of rhesus monkeys to a period of separation from their mothers. *J. Child Psychol. Psychiat.*

Kaufman, I.C. and Rosenblum, L.A. 1969. Effects of separation from mother on the emotional behaviour of infant monkeys. *Ann. NY Acad. Sci.* 159, 681-95

Lorenz, K. 1966. *On Aggression.* London: Methuen

Morris, D. 1967. *The Naked Ape: A Zoologist's Study of the Human Animal.* London: Cape

Rosenblum, L.A. and Kaufman, I.C. 1967. Laboratory observations of early mother/infant relations in pigtail and bonnet macaques. In S. Altmann (ed.), *Social Communication Among Primates.* Chicago: University of Chicago Press, 33-41

Spencer-Booth, Y. and Hinde, R.A. Forthcoming. Effects of six-days separation from mother on 18- 32-week-old rhesus monkeys. *Anim. Behav.*

Van Lawick-Goodall, J. 1968. The behaviour of free-living chimpanzees in the Gombe Stream Reserve. *Anim. Behav. Monographs* 1, 161-311

2 Mother/Infant Relations in Monkeys and Humans: A Reply to Professor Hinde

Bibring, E. 1953. The mechanism of depression. In *Affective Disorders*. New York: International Universities Press, 13-48

Bowlby, J. 1960. Separation anxiety. *Int. J. Psychoanal.* 41, 1

Engel, G.L. and Reichsman, F. 1956. Spontaneous and experimentally induced depressions in an infant with a gastric fistula. A contribution to the problem of depression. *J. Am. Psychoan. Ass.* 4, 428

Engel, G.L. 1962. Anxiety and depression-withdrawal: the primary effects of unpleasure. *Int. J. Psychoanal.* 43, 89

Fleener, D.E. and Cairns, R.B. 1970. Attachment behavior in human infants. *Devel. Psychol.* 2, 215-23

Frank, R.L. 1954. The organized adaptive aspect of the depression-elation response. In Hoch and Zubin (eds.) *Depression*, New York: Grune and Stratton, 51-65

Goodall, J. Van Lawick-. 1965. Chimpanzees of the Gombe Stream Reserve. In I. DeVore (ed.), *Primate Behavior*. New York: Holt, Rinehart and Winston

Heinicke, C.M. and Westheimer, I.J. 1965. *Brief Separations*. New York: International Universities Press

Hess, E.H. 1959. Imprinting. *Science* 130, 133-41

Hinde, R.A., Spencer-Booth Y., and Bruce, M. 1966. Effects of 6-day maternal deprivation on rhesus monkey infants. *Nature* 210, 1021

Kaufman, I.C. and Rosenblum, L.A. A behavioral taxonomy for *Macaca nemestrina* and *Macaca radiata:* based on longitudinal observations of family groups in the laboratory. *Primates* 7, 205-58

Kaufman, I.C. and Rosenblum, L.A. 1967a. Depression in infant monkeys separated from their mothers. *Science* 155, 1030-1

Kaufman, I.C. and Rosenblum, L.A. 1967b. The reaction to separation in infant monkeys: anaclitic depression and conservation-withdrawal. *Psychosom. Med.* 29, 648-75

Kaufman, I.C. and Rosenblum, L.A. 1969. The waning of the mother-infant bond in two species of macaque. In B. Foss (ed.), *Determinants of Infant Behaviour,* vol. 4, London: Methuen

Kaufman, J.H. 1966. Behaviour of infant rhesus monkeys and their mothers in a free-ranging band. *Zoologica* 51, 17-28

Mahler, M.S. and McDevitt, J.B. 1968. Observations on adaptation and defense in statu nascendi. *Psychoanal. Quart.* 37, 1-21

Mason, J.W. 1968. Organization of the multiple endocrine responses to avoidance in the monkey. *Psychosom. Med.* 30, 774

Riss, W. and Scalia, F. 1967. *Functional Pathways of the Central Nervous System.* Amsterdam: Elsevier

Rosenblum, L.A. and Harlow, H.F. 1963. Approach-avoidance conflict in the mother-surrogate situation. *Psychol. Rep.* 12, 83-5

Schneirla, T.C. 1959. An evolutionary and developmental theory of biphasic processes underlying approach and withdrawal. In M.R. Jones (ed.), *Nebraska Symposium on Motivation.* Lincoln: University of Nebraska Press

Seay, B., Hansen, E., and Harlow, H.F. Mother-infant separation in monkeys. *J. Child Psychol. Psychiat.* 3, 123

Seay, B. and Harlow, H.F. 1965. Maternal separation in the rhesus monkey. *J. Nerv. Ment. Dis.* 140, 434

Spitz, R.A. 1945. Hospitalism. *Psychoanal. Stud. Child.* 1, 53

Spitz, R.A. 1946. Anaclitic depression. *Psychoanal. Stud. Child.* 2, 313

Spitz, R.A. 1965. The evolution of dialogue. In M. Schur (ed.), *Drives, Affects, Behavior* 2, 170-90

Washburn, S.L. and Hamburg, D.A. 1965. The implications of primate research. In I. DeVore (ed.), *Primate Behavior.* New York: Holt, Rinehart and Winston

3 Constraints on Learning: Development of Bird Song

Chomsky, N. 1967. The formal nature of language. Appendix A. In E. Lenneberg (ed.), *Biological Foundations of Language*. New York: John Wiley

Foss, B.M. 1964. Mimicry in mynahs (*Gracula religiosa*): a test of Mowrer's theory. *Brit. J. Psychol.* 55, 85-8

Hayes, C. 1951. *The Ape in our House*. New York: Harper and Row

Immelmann, K. 1969. Song development in the zebra finch and other estrildid finches. In R.A. Hinde (ed.), *Bird Vocalizations*. Cambridge: Cambridge University Press

Kellogg, W.N. 1968. Communication and language in the home-raised chimpanzee. *Science* 162, 423-7

Konishi, M. 1964. Effects of deafening on song development in two species of juncos. *Condor* 66, 85-102

Konishi, M. 1965. The role of auditory feedback in the control of vocalization in the white-crowned sparrow. *Z. Tierpsychol.* 22, 770-83

Konishi, M. and Nottebohm, F. 1969. Experimental studies in the ontogency of avian vocalizations. In R.A. Hinde (ed.), *Bird Vocalizations*

Lenneberg, E.H. 1967. *Biological Foundations of Language*. New York: John Wiley

Lorenz, K. 1950. The comparative method in studying innate behaviour patterns. *Symp. Soc. Exp. Biol.* 4, 221-68

Lorenz, K. 1965. *Evolution and Modification of Behavior*. Chicago: University of Chicago Press

Marler, P. 1963. Inheritance and learning in the development of animal vocalizations. In R.G. Busnel (ed.), *Acoustic Behavior of Animals*. Amsterdam: Elsevier

Marler, P. 1970. A comparative approach to vocal development: song learning in the white-crowned sparrow. *J. Comp. Physiol. Psychol.* 71, 1-25

Marler, P. and Mundinger, P. Forthcoming. Vocal learning in birds. In H. Moltz (ed.), *The Ontogeny of Vertebrate Behavior*. New York: Academic Press

Mowrer, O.H. 1950. On the psychology of 'talking birds' − a contribution to language and personality theory. In O.H. Mowrer (ed.), *Learning Theory and Personality Dynamics*. New York: Ronald Press

Mowrer, O.H. 1958. Hearing and speaking: an analysis of language learning. *J. Speech Hearing Dis.* 23, 143-52

Mulligan, J.A. 1966. Singing behavior and its development in the song sparrow, *Melospiza melodia*. Berkeley: *University of California Publ. Zool.* 81, 1-76

Mundinger, P.C. 1970. Vocal imitation and individual recognition of finch calls. *Science* 168, 480-2

Nicolai, J. 1959. Familientradition in der Gesangsentwicklung des Gimpels (*Pyrrhula pyrrhula* L.). *J. Ornith.* 100, 39-46

Nottebohm, F. 1970. Ontogeny of bird song. *Science* 167, 950-6

Nottebohm, F. Forthcoming. Neural lateralization of vocal control in a passerine bird. I. Song. *J. Exp. Zool.*

Nottebohm, F. Forthcoming. Neural lateralization of vocal control in a passerine bird. II. Subsong, calls, and a theory of vocal learning. *Ibid.*

Thorpe, W.H. 1955. Comments on the *Bird Fancyer's Delight,* together with notes on imitation in the sub-song of the chaffinch. *Ibis* 97, 247-51

Thorpe, W.H. 1961. *Bird Song: The Biology of Vocal Communication and Expression in Birds.* Cambridge: Cambridge University Press

WILLIAM A. MASON, SUZANNE D. HILL,
CURTIS E. THOMSEN

4 Perceptual Aspects of Filial Attachment in Monkeys

Harlow, H.F. and Zimmermann, R.R. 1958. The development of affectional
   responses in infant monkeys. *Proc. Am. Phil. Soc.* 102, 501-9
Mason, W.A., Hill, S.D., and Thomsen, C.E. Forthcoming. Perceptual factors
   in the development of filial attachment. In *Proceedings of the Third
   Congress of the International Primatological Society*

5 Some Features of Early Behavioural Development in Kittens

Fuller, J.L., Easler, C.A., and Banks, E.M. 1950. Formation of conditioned avoidance responses in young puppies. *Amer. J. Physiol.* 2, 277-80

James, W.T., and Cannon, D.J. 1952. Conditioned avoiding response in puppies. *Ibid.* 168, 251-3

Koepke, J.E. and Pribram, K.H. 1971. Effect of milk on the maintenance of sucking in kittens from birth to six months. *J. Comp. Physiol. Psychol.* 75, 363-77

Lipsitt, L.P. 1967. Learning in the human infant. In H.W. Stevenson, E.H. Hess, and H.L. Rheingold (eds.), *Early Behavior and Developmental Approaches.* New York: Wiley, 255-7

Mason, W.A. and Harlow, H.F. 1958. Formation of conditioned responses in infant monkeys. *J. Comp. Physiol. Psychol.* 51, 68-70

Rheingold, H.L. and Eckerman, C.O. 1971. Familiar social and nonsocial stimuli and the kitten's response to a strange environment. *Devel. Psychobiol.* 4, 71-89

Rosenblatt, J.S. 1971. Suckling and home orientation in the kitten: a comparative developmental study. In E. Tobach (ed.), *Biopsychology of Development.* New York: Academic Press

Rosenblatt, J.S., Turkewitz, G., and Schneirla, T.C. 1961. Early socialization in the domestic cat as based on feeding and other relationships between female and young. In B.F. Foss, (ed.), *Determinants of Infant Behaviour.* London: Methuen, 51-74

Rosenblatt, J.S., Turkewitz, G., and Schneirla, T.C. 1969. Development of home orientation in newly born kittens. *Trans. NY Acad. Sci.* 31, 231-50

Schneirla, T.C. and Rosenblatt, J.S. 1961. Behavioral organization and genesis of the social bond in insects and mammals. *Am. J. Orthopsychiat.* 31, 223-53

Schneirla, T.C. and Rosenblatt, J.S. 1963. Critical periods in the development of behavior. *Science* 139, 1110-15

Schneirla, T.C., Rosenblatt, J.S., and Tobach, E. 1963. Maternal behavior in the cat. In H.L. Rheingold (ed.), *Maternal Behavior in Mammals.* New York: Wiley, 122-68

Scott, J.P. 1958. Critical periods in the development of social behavior in puppies. *Psychosom. Med.* 20, 42-54

Scott, J.P., 1962. Critical periods in behavioral development. *Science* 138, 945-58

Stanley, W.C., Bacon, W.H., and Fehr, C. 1970. Discriminated instrumental learning in neonatal dogs. *J. Comp. Physiol. Psychol.* 70, 335-43

Thoman, E., Wetzel, A., and Levine, S. 1968. Learning in the neonatal rat. *Anim. Behav.* 16, 54-7

IRVEN DEVORE, MELVIN J. KONNER

6 Infancy
in Hunter-Gatherer Life:
An Ethological Perspective

Ardrey, R. 1961. *African Genesis*. New York: Atheneum
Ardrey, R. 1966. *The Territorial Imperative*. New York: Atheneum
Ardrey, R. 1970. *The Social Contract*. New York: Atheneum
Blurton-Jones, N.G. (ed.). 1972. *Ethological Studies of Child Behaviour*.
    Cambridge: Cambridge University Press
Bowlby, J. 1953. *Child Care and the Growth of Love*. London: the White-
    friars Press, Ltd
Bowlby, J. (ed.). 1966. *Maternal Care and Mental Health; A report prepared
    on behalf of the World Health Organization as a contribution to the
    United Nations program for the welfare of homeless children*. New York:
    Schocken Books
Bowlby, J. 1969. *Attachment and Loss,* vol. I. London: Hogarth
Draper, P. 1972. !Kung Bushman childhood in an ecological framework.
    PhD thesis, Harvard University, Cambridge, Mass.
Eibl-Eibesfeldt, I. 1970. *Ethology: The Biology of Behavior*. New York: Holt,
    Rinehart and Winston
Erikson, E.H. 1950. *Childhood and Society*. New York: Norton
Freud, S. 1920. *Introductory Lectures to Psychoanalysis*. New York: Boni
    and Liveright
Hamburg, D.A. 1963. Emotions in the perspective of human evolution. In
    P.H. Knapp (ed.), *Expression of the Emotions in Man*. New York: Inter-
    national Universities Press
Harlow, H.F. 1962. Social deprivation in monkeys. *Scientific American* 207
    (5), 136-46
Harlow, H.F. and Harlow, M.K. 1969. Effects of various mother-infant rela-
    tionships on rhesus monkey behaviors. In B.M. Foss (ed.), *Determinants of
    Infant Behavior,* vol. 4. London: Methuen
Konner, M.J. 1972. Aspects of the developmental ethology of a foraging
    people. In N.G. Blurton-Jones (1972)
Lee, R.B. 1965. *Subsistence ecology of the !Kung*. PhD thesis, University of
    California, Berkeley. Ann Arbor, Michigan: University Microfilms
Lee, R.B. 1968. What hunters do for a living, or, how to make out on scarce
    resources. In R.B. Lee and I. DeVore (1968)
Lee, R.B. 1969. !Kung Bushman subsistence: an input-output analysis.
    National Museums of Canada Bulletin 230. Contributions to anthro-
    pology: ecological essays

Lee, R.B. 1972. The !Kung Bushmen of Botswana. In M.G. Bicchieri (ed.), *Hunters and Gatherers Today.* New York: Holt, Rinehart, Winston

Lee, R.B., and DeVore, I. (eds.). 1968. *Man the Hunter.* Chicago: Aldine

Lee, R.B. and DeVore, I. (eds.). 1974. *Kalahari Hunter-Gatherers.* Cambridge: Harvard University Press

Levine, R.A. 1970. Cross-cultural study in child psychology. In P.H. Mussen (ed.), *Carmichael's Manual of Child Psychology.* New York: John Wiley and Sons

Lockhard, R.B. 1971. Reflections on the fall of comparative psychology: is there a message for us all? *American Psychologist* 26 (2), 168-79

Lorenz, K. 1966. *On Aggression.* New York: Harcourt, Brace and World

Mead, M. 1966. A cultural anthropologist's approach to maternal deprivation. In Bowlby (1966)

Morris, D. (ed.). 1967. *Primate Ethology.* Chicago: Aldine

Morris, D. 1968. *The Naked Ape.* New York: McGraw-Hill

Prechtl, H.F.R. and Beintema, D.J. 1964. *The Neurological Examination of the Full-term Newborn Infant.* London: Heinemann

Radcliffe-Brown, A.R. 1931. Social organization of Australian tribes. *Oceania Monographs,* I

Rafael, D. 1971. Effects of supportive behavior on location. Paper presented at the meeting of the American Anthropological Association, New York (Nov.) 1971

Sahlins, M. 1968. Discussions, Part II 9b. In Lee and DeVore (1968)

Service, E.R. 1966. *The Hunters.* Englewood Cliffs, NJ: Prentice-Hall

Spock, B. 1968. *Baby and Child Care.* New revised and enlarged edition. New York: Pocket Books

Trivers, R.L. 1972. Parental investment and sexual selection. In Bernard Campbell (ed.), *Sexual Selection and the Descent of Man 1877-1971.* Chicago: Aldine

Whiting, John W.M. 1961. Socialization process and personality. In F.L.K. Hsu (ed.), *Psychological Anthropology.* Homewood, Ill.: The Dorsey Press

JOHN HURRELL CROOK

7 Social Organization
and the Developmental Environment

Aldrich-Blake, F.P.G. 1970. Problems of social structure in forest monkeys. In J.H. Crook (ed.), *Social Behaviour in Birds and Mammals.* London: Academic Press

Aldrich-Blake, F.P.G. 1970. The ecology and behaviour of the Blue Monkey (*Cercopithecus mitis stuhlmani*). Doctoral thesis, Bristol University library

Bernstein, I.S. 1966. Analysis of a key role in a capuchin (*Cebus albifrans*) group. *Tulane. Stud. Zool.* 13 (2), 49-54

Burton, F. 1971. Personal communication

Crook, J.H. 1970. Social behaviour and ethology. In Crook (ed.), *Social Behaviour in Birds and Mammals*

Crook, J.H. 1970a. The socio-ecology of primates. In Crook (ed.), *Social Behaviour in Birds and Mammals*

Crook, J.H. Forthcoming. Sexual selection, dimorphism and social organization in the primates

Crook, J.H. and Gartlan, J.S. 1966. Evolution of primate societies *Nature* 210, 1200-3

Deag, J. and Crook, J.H. 1971. Social behaviour and agonistic buffering in the wild Barbary, *Macaca sylvana L. Folia Primat.* (in press)

Espinas, A. 1878. *Des sociétés animales.* Paris: Baillière

Gartlan, J.S. 1970. Personal communication

Gautier, J.P. and Gauthier-Hion, A. 1969. Les associations polyspecifiques chez les Cercopithecidae du Gabon. *La Terre et la vie* 2, 164-201

Hall, K.R.L. 1966. Behaviour and ecology of the wild Patas monkey, *Erythrocebus patas,* in Uganda. *J. Zool.* 148, 158-87

Hall, K.R.L. and DeVore, I. 1965. Baboon social behaviour. In I. DeVore (ed.), *Primate Behaviour.* New York: Holt, Rinehart and Winston

Hall, K.R.L. and Mayer, B. 1967. Social interactions in a group of captive Patas monkeys (*Erythrocebus patas*). *Folia Primat.* 5, 213-36

Harlow, H.F. and Harlow, M.K. 1962. Social deprivation in monkeys. *Sci. Am.* 207 (5), 137-46

Hinde, R.A. and Spencer-Booth, Y. 1967. The behaviour of socially living rhesus monkeys in their first two and a half years. *Anim. Behav.* 15, 169-96

Huxley, J.S. 1923. Courtship activities in the Red Throated Diver (*Colymbus stellatus* portopp) together with a discussion of the evolution of courtship in birds. *J. Linn. Soc.* 35, 253-92

Itani, J. 1959. Paternal care in the wild Japanese monkey, *Macaca f. fuscata*. *Primates* 2, 61-93

Jay, P. 1965. The common langur of N. India. In DeVore (ed.), *Primate Behaviour*

Jolly, C.J. 1969. The seed eaters: a new model of hominid differentiation based on a baboon analogy. *Man* 5 (1) (March), 5-26

Kummer, H. 1967. Tripartite relations in Hamadryas baboons. In S.A. Altmann (ed.), *Social Communication among primates*. Chicago: University of Chicago Press

Mason, W.A. 1965. The social development of monkeys and apes. In DeVore (ed.), *Primate Behavior*

Michael, R. and Keverne, B. 1968. Pheromones in the communication of sexual status in Primates. *Nature* 218, 746-9

Michael, R. and Keverne, B. 1970. Primate sex pheromones of vaginal origin. *Ibid.* 225, 84-5

Mizuhara, H. 1969. Social changes of Japanese monkey troops in the Takasakiyama. *Primates* 5, 27-52

Petrucci, R. 1906. Origine polyphylétique, homotypie et non-comparabilité directe des sociétés animales. *Instituts Solvay. Travaux de l'Institute de Sociologie. Notes et memoires* Fasc. 7, Bruxelles: Mich. et thou.

Reynolds, V. 1970. Roles and role change in monkey society: the consort relationship of rhesus monkeys. *Man* 5 (3), 449-65

Rowell, T.E., Hinde, R.A., and Spencer-Booth, Y. 1964. Aunt-infant interaction in captive rhesus groups. *Anim. Behav.* 12, 219-26

Sugiyama, Y. 1960. On the division of a natural troop of Japanese monkeys at Takasakiyama. *Primates* 2, 109-44

Sugiyama, Y. 1967. Social Organization of *Hanuman* Langurs. In Altmann (ed.), *Social Communication among Primates*. Chicago: Univ. Chicago Press

Struhsaker, T.T. and Gartlan, J.S. 1970. Observations on the behaviour and ecology of the Patas monkey (*Erythrocebus patas*) in the Waza reserve, Cameroon. *J. Zool.* 161, 49-63

Vandenbergh, J.G. 1967. The development of social structure in free-ranging rhesus monkeys. *Behaviour* 29, 179-94

Wilson, A.P. 1968. Social behaviour of free ranging rhesus monkeys with an emphasis on aggression. Doctoral thesis, University of California, Berkeley

WILLIAM A. MASON

8 Differential Grouping Patterns in Two Species of South American Monkey

Alvarez, F. 1968. Effects of sex hormones on the social organization of the squirrel monkey, *Saimiri sciureus*. Unpublished doctoral dissertation, Tulane University

Castell, R. and Ploog, D. 1967. Zum Socialverhalten der Totenkopf-Affen (*Saimiri sciureus*): Auseninandersetzung zwischen zwei Kolonien. *Z. Tierpsychol.* 24, 625-41

Mason, W.A. 1966. Social organization of the South American monkey, *Callicebus moloch:* a preliminary report. *Tulane Stud. Zool.* 13, 23-8

Mason, W.A. 1968. Use of space by Callicebus groups. In P.C. Jay (ed.), *Primates: Studies in Adaptation and Variability.* New York: Holt, Rinehart and Winston

Mason, W.A. and Epple, G. 1969. Social organization in experimental groups of *Saimiri* and *Callicebus*. In C.R. Carpenter (ed.), *Proceedings of the Second International Congress of Primatology,* vol. 1. Basel: S. Karger, 59-65

Rosenblum, L.A., Levy, E.J., and Kaufman, I.C. 1968. Social behaviour of squirrel monkeys and the reaction to strangers. *Anim. Behav.* 16, 288-93

Thorington, R.W., Jr. 1967. Feeding and activity of *Cebus* and *Saimiri* in a Colombian forest. In D. Starck, R. Schneider, and H.J. Kuhn (eds.), *Progress in Primatology.* Stuttgart: Gustav Fischer Verlag, 180-4

Thorington, R.W., Jr. 1968. Observations of squirrel monkeys in a Colombian forest. In L.A. Rosenblum and R.W. Cooper (eds.), *The Squirrel Monkey.* New York: Academic Press, 69-85

9 Comparative Ethology and the Evolution of Behaviour

Andrew, R.J. 1956. Intention movements of flight in certain passerines, and their use in systematics. *Behaviour* 10, 179-204

Atz, J.W. 1970. The application of the idea of homology to behaviour. In L.R. Aronson, E. Tobach, D.S. Lehrman and J.S. Rosenblatt (eds.), *Development and Evolution of Behavior.* San Francisco: Freeman

Blest, A.D. 1957. The evolution of protective displays in the Saturnioidea and Sphingidae (Lepidoptera). *Behaviour* 11, 257-309

Blest, A.D. 1961. The concept of ritualization. In W.H. Thorpe and O.L. Zangwill (eds.), *Current Problems in Animal Behaviour.* Cambridge: Cambridge University press

Daanje, A. 1954. On locomotory movements in birds and the intention movements derived from them. *Behaviour* 3, 48-98

Darwin, C.R. 1859. *The Origin of Species.* New York: Appleton

Hinde, R.A. and Tinbergen, N. 1958. The comparative study of species-specific behavior. In A. Roe and G.G. Simpson (eds.), *Behavior and Evolution.* New Haven: Yale University Press

Kaplan, A. 1964. *The Conduct of Inquiry.* San Francisco: Chandler

Lorenz, K. 1935. Der Kumpan in der Unwelt des Vogels. *J.F. Ornith.* 83, 137-213, 289-413

Lorenz, K. 1941. Vergleichende Bewegungssudien an Anatinen. *Suppl. J. Ornith.* 89, 194-294

Lorenz, K. 1950. The comparative method in studying innate behaviour patterns. *Symp. Soc. Exp. Biol.* 4, 221-68

Lorenz, K. 1965. *Evolution and Modification of Behavior.* Chicago: University of Chicago Press

Lorenz, K. 1966. *On Aggression.* London: Methuen

Morris, D. 1957. 'Typical intensity' and its relation to the problems of ritualization. *Behaviour* 11, 1-12

Russel, E.S. 1916. *Form and Function.* London: John Murray

Schmidt, R.S. 1958. The nests of *Apicotermes tragardhi;* new evidence on the evolution of nest-building. *Behaviour* 12, 76-94

Tinbergen, N. 1951. *The Study of Instinct.* Oxford: Oxford University Press

Tinbergen, N. 1952. 'Derived' activities, their causation, biological significance and emancipation during evolution. *Quart. Rev. Biol.* 27, 1-32

Tinbergen, N. 1959. Comparative studies of the behaviour of gulls (Laridae): a progress report. *Behaviour* 15, 1-70

ERNST W. HANSEN

10 Some Aspects of Behavioural Development in Evolutionary Perspective

deBeer, G.R. 1940. *Embryos and Ancestors.* Oxford: Clarendon

Clark, W.E. le Gross 1959. *The Antecedents of Man.* Chicago: Quadrangle

Crook, J.H. 1970. Social organization and the environment. *Anim. Behav.* 18, 197-208

Crook, J.H. and Gartlan, J.S. 1966. Evolution of primate societies. *Nature* 210, 1200

Eibl-Eibesfeldt, I. 1970. *Ethology: The Biology of Behavior.* New York: Holt, Rinehart, and Winston

Hamburg, D.A. 1968. Emotions in the perspective of human evolution. In S.L. Washburn and Phyllis Jay (eds.), *Perspectives on Human Evolution.* New York: Holt, Rinehart, and Winston

Hamburg, D.A. 1968. Evolution of emotional responses: evidence from recent research on nonhuman primates. *Sci. & Psychoanal.* 12, 39-54

Harlow, H.F. and Harlow, M.K. 1965. The affectional systems. In A.H. Schrier, H.F. Harlow, and F. Stollnitz (eds.), *Behavior of Nonhuman Primates.* New York: Academic Press

Harlow, H.F. and Harlow, M.K. 1969. Effects of various mother-infant relationships on rhesus monkey behaviors. In B.M. Foss (ed.), *Determinants of Infant Behavior.* London: Methuen

Mason, W.A. 1968. Early social deprivation in the nonhuman primates: implications for human behavior. In D.C. Glass (ed.), *Environmental Influences.* New York: Rockefeller University Press

Schultz, A.H. 1968. The recent hominoid primates. In S.L. Washburn and Phyllis C. Jay (eds.), *Perspectives on Human Evolution.* New York: Holt, Rinehart, and Winston

DANIEL S. LEHRMAN

11 Can Psychiatrists use Ethology?

Bowlby, J. 1969. *Attachment.* New York: Basic Books
Hinde, R.A. 1970. *Animal Behavior.* 2nd ed. New York: McGraw-Hill
Lorenz, K. 1970. *Studies in Animal and Human Behaviour,* vols. 1 and 2. Cambridge, Mass.: Harvard University Press
Mead, M. 1928. *Coming of Age in Samoa.* New York: William Morrow
Spencer-Booth, Y. and Hinde, R.A. 1967. The effects of separating rhesus monkey infants from their mothers for six days. *Journal of Child Psychology and Psychiatry* 7, 179-97
Tinbergen, N. 1951. *The Study of Instinct.* Oxford: Oxford University Press

HARRY F. HARLOW

12   Induction and Alleviation of Depressive States in Monkeys

Bowlby, J. 1969. *Attachment.* New York: Basic Books

Harlow, H.F. 1958. The nature of love. *American Psychologist* 13, 673-85

Harlow, H.F. and Harlow, M.K. 1962. Social deprivation in monkeys. *Sci. Am.* 207, 136-46

Harlow, H.F., Suomi, S.J., and McKinney, W.T. 1970. Experimental production of depression in monkeys. *Mainly Monkeys* 1, 6-12

Seay, B., Hansen, E. and Harlow, H.F. 1962. Mother-infant separation in monkeys. *J. Child Psychol. Psychiat.* 3, 123-32

Suomi, S.J., Harlow, H.F., and Domek, C.J. 1970. Effect of repetitive infant-infant separation of young monkeys. *J. Abnormal Psychol.* 76, 161-72

13 Ethological Perspectives on Human Aggressive Behaviour

Altmann, S.A. 1967. *Social Communication Among Primates.* Chicago: University of Chicago Press, 392

Ardrey, R. 1966. *The Territorial Imperative.* New York: Atheneum

Bandura, A. 1965. In Leonard Berkowitz (ed.), *Advances in Experimental Social Psychology.* vol. II. New York: Academic Press

Campbell, D.T. 1965. Ethnocentric and other altruistic motives. In D. Levine (ed.), *Nebraska Symposium on Motivation.* Lincoln: University of Nebraska Press

Clayton, R.B., Kogura, J., and Kraemer, H.C. 1970. *Nature* 226, 810

Crook, J.H. 1968. In M.F.A. Montagu (ed.), *Man and Aggression.* Oxford: Oxford University Press, 141

DeVore, I. and Hall, K.R.L. 1965. In I. DeVore (ed.), *Primate Behavior: Field Studies of Monkeys and Apes.* New York: Holt, Rinehart and Winston, 20

Hall, K.R.L., and DeVore, I. 1965. In DeVore (ed.), *Primate Behavior: Field Studies of Monkeys and Apes,* 53

Hamburg, D.A. 1969. Observations of mother-infant interactions in primate field studies. In B.M. Foss (ed.), *Determinants of Infant Behavior,* IV. London: Methuen, 3

Hinde, R. 1967. *New Society.* March 2, 302

Lorenz, K. 1966. *On Aggression.* New York: Harcourt, Brace, World

Money, J. and Ehrhardt, A.A. 1968. In R.P. Michael (ed.), *Endocrinology and Human Behavior.* New York: Oxford University Press, 32

Montagu, M.F.A. (ed.). 1968. *Man and Aggression.* New York: Oxford University Press

Morris, D. 1967. *The Naked Ape.* New York: McGraw-Hill

Morris, D. 1969. *The Human Zoo.* New York: McGraw-Hill

Ransom, T. 1971. *Ecology and Social Behavior of Baboons at the Gombe National Park.* PhD dissertation, University of California, Berkeley

Riopelle, A. 1960. In R. Wattes, D. Rethingshater, and W. Caldwell (eds.), *Principles of Comparative Psychology.* New York: McGraw-Hill

Rowell, T.E. 1967. *Anim. Behav.* 15, 499

Sackett, G.P. 1966. *Science* 154, 1468

Southwick, C.H. 1969. Aggressive behavior of rhesus monkeys in natural and captive groups. In S. Garattini and E.B. Sigg (eds.), *Aggressive Behavior.* New York: John Wiley and Sons

Storr, A. 1968. *Human Aggression.* New York: Atheneum

van Lawick-Goodall, Jane. 1968. Expressive movements and communication in free-ranging chimpanzees: a preliminary report. In P.C. Jay (ed.), *Primates: Studies in Adaptation and Variability*. New York: Holt Rinehart and Winston, 53

Washburn, S.L. and Hamburg, D.A. 1968. Aggressive behavior in old world monkeys and apes. In Jay (ed.), *Primates: Studies in Adaptation and Variability*, 458-78

Young, W., Goy, R., and Phoenix, C. 1964. *Science* 143, 212

Zimbardo, P.G. 1969. The human choice: individuation, reason, and order versus deindividuation, impulse, and chaos. In W.J. Arnold (ed.), *Nebraska Symposium on Motivation*. Lincoln: University of Nebraska Press 237-307

Index

49362